MW00618315

# The Fellowship of the River

# THE FELLOWSHIP
# OF THE RIVER

A Medical Doctor's Exploration into Traditional
Amazonian Plant Medicine

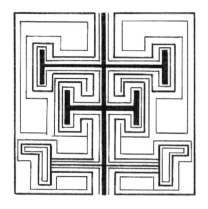

## Joseph Tafur, MD
Foreword by Gabor Maté, MD

This edition first published in 2017 by Espiritu Books
10645 N. Tatum Blvd., Ste. 200-283
Phoenix, AZ 85028
espiritubooks@gmail.com

Copyright © 2017 Joe Tafur
Foreword Copyright © 2017 Gabriel Maté
All rights reserved. No part of this publication may be reproduced or transmitted in any form or by any means without permission in writing from Joseph Tafur and Espiritu Books.

Espiritu Books
Edited by Caroline Pincus (carolinepincus.com)
Cover art and chapter drawings by Markus Drassl
Cover design by Jane Hagaman and Andrea Contreras
Text design by Jane Hagaman

ISBN: 978-0-9986095-0-8

Printed by CreateSpace

*for my father*

# Contents

# Note

To see the many photos and images related to this book, please visit my website: https://drjoetafur.com/the-fellowship-of-the-river/.

# Disclaimer

The material presented in this book is intended for informational purposes only, not to diagnose, prescribe, or treat a health concern or ailment. If you are concerned about your health, please seek advice from a professional in your area.

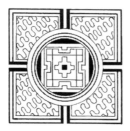

# Foreword

As a Western-trained doctor, I have long been aware of modern medicine's limitations in handling chronic conditions of mind and body. For all our astonishing achievements, there are a host of ailments whose ravages we physicians can at best alleviate. In our narrow pursuit of cure, we fail to comprehend the essence of healing. Hence the popularity of ayahuasca, the Amazonian plant medicine to which many Westerners are turning to heal from physical illness or mental anguish, or as they seek a sense of meaning amid the growing alienation in our culture.

Ayahuasca and plant healing is the subject of this work by my Colombian-American medical colleague Joe Tafur. Dr. Tafur's book serves a triple function: a fascinating personal history of shamanic self-discovery, a compendium of convincing case histories of the plant's healing potential, and an informed scientific meditation on how this jungle vine and related plants can, under shamanic guidance, result in the astonishing physical, emotional, and spiritual transformations he has witnessed, as have I, in our work with the madre—"the mother," as the vine is called in the Amazon basin.

One of the most frustrating failures of Western medical practice is its lack of awareness of the unity of mind and body *despite* voluminous, elegant, and absolutely persuasive research evidence that the distinction between mind and body is false, unscientific, and—in real life—impossible. Joe Tafur relies adeptly on such evidence to indicate why the "miracles" he describes arising from shamanic plant ceremonies are, in fact, precisely what one would expect if one were grounded in a holistic understanding of human beings in health and illness.

His triumphant case histories include relief from chronic conditions that mainstream medical practice considers subject at best to symptom management, but never cure: psoriasis, chronic migraine, inflammatory bowel disease, along with mental health conditions such as depression and anxiety.

The employment of ayahuasca in the treatment of refractory mental health issues has long been studied, in the countries where official paranoia and narrow-mindedness have not interdicted the treatment with the plant and where its use is grounded in indigenous cultural traditions. As an article in *The Medical Post* reported, "[in] a review of 28 human studies recently published in the *Journal of Psychopharmacology*, the researchers concluded that not only did the ayahuasca experience show 'anti-depressive and anti-addictive potentials,' it also had a physiological effect on the brain, affecting the size and thickness of the areas associated with impulse control, decision-making, pain and memory.'" These are, of course, some of the key brain systems impaired in addictions.

From my own very first experience with ayahuasca, I saw very clearly how it can help people with emotional and spiritual issues. It opened me up, allowed me to experience emotions of sadness and loss I had long suppressed, but also a deep love that was greater than any grief or trauma I had experienced. Brain scans show that it activates parts of the cerebrum where childhood emotional memories are stored, and also areas where adult insight is generated.

In its proper ceremonial setting, under compassionate and experienced guidance, the plant—or, as tradition has it, the spirit of the plant—puts people in touch with their repressed pain and trauma, the very factors that drive all dysfunctional mind states. Consciously experiencing our primal pain loosens its hold on us. Thus may ayahuasca achieve in a few sittings what many years of psychotherapy can only aspire to. It also allows people to re-experience long-lost inner qualities, such as wholeness, trust, love, and a sense of possibility. People quite literally remember themselves.

But how does the plant support healing from conditions such as chronic inflammatory bowel disease or psoriasis, or other auto-immune conditions, as both Joe Tafur and I have observed? Dr. Tafur's experience and theoretical explorations provide a more-than-plausible exploration of that question.

Unlike the prevailing Western mind-body split, a holistic understanding informs many aboriginal wisdom teachings. Like all plant-based indigenous practices around the world, the use of ayahuasca arises from a tradition where mind and body are seen as inseparable, in sickness and in health. Here Joe Tafur relies on impeccable Western science theories about the plant's healing capacities—science that has amply confirmed the ancient wisdom.

In several chapters Dr. Tafur explains, and with case examples illuminates, the unity of mind/body in health and illness. He shows how emotional trauma can cause inflammation of, say, the lung's airways or other organs; how emotional disturbance can dysregulate the autonomic nervous system; how stress impairs and confuses the body's immune apparatus. It follows that a regaining of emotional balance, the working out of past trauma, and connection with our deeper humanity should and can have powerfully beneficial physiological effects. Such experiential transformation, if genuine, can powerfully affect the hormonal apparatus, the nervous and immune systems, and all organs such as the brain, the gut, and the heart. Hence ayahuasca's potential healing capacity.

As Dr. Tafur writes, "Reconnecting to your bodily senses also involves reconnecting the mind to your internal sensations: how you feel inside your body, your heart, your gut, and throughout. This sense is called interoception. We experience our emotions through these sensations. These internal sensations also inform us about the physiologic condition of our body." Again, we remember ourselves.

The new science of epigenetics has shown that emotional stressors can have negative effects on gene functioning, effects that are transmittable even to future generations. Tafur also speculates, quite plausibly, that positive experiences can help to reverse such changes or, indeed, induce positive changes in gene activity.

As Tafur scrupulously points out, it is not all good news. Ayahuasca can be exploited for financial gain by unscrupulous or just inexperienced practitioners or even for the sexual gratification of healers preying on vulnerable clients, most often young females. Such cases are notorious in the ayahuasca world, as are shamanic infighting, hexing, and power struggles. One must find the right context to be exposed to such a potentially powerful modality—hence Joe Tafur's own work to establish a healing center in Peru, the Nihue Rao Centro Espiritual, and hence my own work leading plant retreats, and hence also The Temple of the Way of Light, also in Peru.

Nor is the plant a panacea. People with certain mental health conditions, such as mania or psychosis, for example, must avoid it. More generally, the plant opens pathways for many but the healing is far from complete with such openings. As I have learned and as Joe Tafur carefully advises, processing, integration, and long-term practice must follow the psychedelic experience for the full benefits to accrue. "Open-minded spiritual practices like meditation," he writes, "are a more stable pathway to expanded consciousness. As there are continued stresses, the mind will need continued maintenance . . . Without some form of integration, emotional support and/or new behavior, even the most enlightening psychedelic experience will wane into a mere temporary shift in thinking. However, in the short term, such an experience may give someone the boost they need to find a more stable path."

That boost, however, can be potent and, for many people, absolutely life changing. With this fascinating account of his personal journey and his depiction of healing experiences observed through the eyes of a conservatively trained medical practitioner, Dr. Tafur brings us a long way towards bridging the seemingly incompatible worlds of traditional shamanic healing and Western medical practice.

—*Gabor Maté, MD*
*Fall 2016*

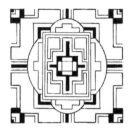

# CHAPTER 1

# The Fellowship of the River

The road was once a river and that's why it's still hungry.

—Ben Okri, *The Famished Road*

Have you ever gone to the doctor for something you were concerned about, and then been told "everything's fine, it's all in your head"? Well, sometimes it is all just in your head, and other times, it's something more. I remember going to the doctor when I was in medical school. I hadn't been feeling well and had some rather vague, subjective complaints. Most of all, I was worried about my breathing, my lungs felt stiff, and I couldn't take a deep breath. The doctor examined me, then ordered a chest x-ray and a few labs. Objectively, everything turned out to be within normal limits. He told me that I had "medical school syndrome" and not to worry too much about it. Although this was somewhat comforting to hear, I didn't feel any better. My problem was beyond the scope of blood tests and x-rays. I was soul sick, spiritually ill. In our brief visit, the doctor didn't ask me too many questions about how I felt inside, in my heart. I can't blame him. Most likely, he wasn't trained to consider those things.

I should know, I'm a medical doctor. But first, I am a living human being, and as it turns out my breathing problems were related to my

1

mental health. I was depressed in medical school. To get better, I would need to venture outside the confines of established medical care. I needed spiritual healing.

Once I found it, my mind calmed and my breathing improved, and I realized that I needed to learn more about spiritual healing. When the time came, I left my books and papers behind and travelled to the Amazon rainforest. I spent years working and training in the Amazon. My traditional education there guided me to a broader understanding of health and disease. This new perspective respects modern biochemistry, anatomy and pharmacology, but it also recognizes the profound influence of the immaterial in medicine, the emotional and spiritual dimensions of health. This is a book about the intersection between biology, emotion, and spirituality. In order to share this new perspective, I will weave my theories into a series of stories, stories about my journey into shamanism.

My interest in heading to the Amazon was in part driven by my desire to understand at a deeper level the depression that had overtaken me during my medical training. Med school had given me professional knowledge, skills, and competencies; but it had also brought me to my knees.

Like many others, my Western medical training left me rather traumatized. To get through it, I needed help. And despite my initial skepticism about psychedelics, I discovered a powerful ally in the plant medicine peyote (see Chapter 4 for more about my experience with peyote). Deep in the Arizona desert, peyote helped me to quiet my mind and reconnect to my heart. My experience in the desert left me very curious about shamanic plant medicine and psychedelic medicines in general.

After medical school, during my residency training, I continued to be interested in a variety of medical traditions and had further encounters with indigenous healing.

After completing residency, I travelled for the first time to the Amazon in 2007. I flew to Iquitos, Peru with my good friend and colleague Keyvan (pronounced Cave-on). Keyvan and I, coincidentally, had paralleled each other through school: University of California,

Los Angeles (UCLA) for college, University of California, San Diego (UCSD) for medical school, and UCLA again for residency in family medicine. For over a decade, Keyvan and I had endured the prescribed program of Western medical training. By the time we had completed our residency, we were ready for something more adventurous. After residency, one can continue medical training in fellowship, such as a Sports Medicine Fellowship or Geriatrics Fellowship. We decided, for fun, that we would create our own fellowship, what Keyvan dubbed the Fellowship of the River (the Amazon River, that is). That first trip exposed me to Traditional Amazonian Plant Medicine (TAPM) and the mysterious world of ayahuasca shamanism.

I had read about ayahuasca and knew that it was considered a sacred plant medicine in the Amazon rainforest, widely revered for its ability to induce powerful visions.

Our five-week Fellowship of the River started with an amazing ayahuasca ceremony at a traditional healing center outside of Iquitos. After our incredible experiences there, we cruised down the Amazon to Brazil and, as planned, we made it to the beach. After our adventure was complete, it was time to head home and start our medical careers. For me, though, the Fellowship of the River wasn't over. It was just beginning.

Shortly afterward, I started postdoctoral research at the UCSD Dept. of Psychiatry, at a lab focused on mind-body medicine. On a break, I returned to Iquitos alone for more traditional plant medicine and more ayahuasca ceremony. After that second visit, the Fellowship of the River took a course of its own. It became the next phase of my medical training. I returned to the Amazon again and again. At first I wasn't entirely sure where it was all guiding me, I was simply following up on my curiosity. But life had other plans for me.

I had become a doctor because I had always wanted to be a healer. Ayahuasca opened my eyes to the world of spiritual healing.

In 2009, two years after the first trip with Keyvan, I started bringing groups down to Iquitos, both to guide others to traditional ayahuasca shamanism and to experience it at a deeper level myself. During these trips, I spent more time with indigenous shamans, and

I saw more and more people benefit from their deep healing practices. As a doctor, I was impressed by the use of sacred plants as a system of medicine and by the profound results. I began to entertain the possibility of training as an ayahuasca shaman.

Over time, I developed a close relationship with a master *ayahuasquero,* Ricardo Amaringo. I first met Ricardo on the original fellowship journey in 2007, and over the years, I had helped him with translation and we became friends. He was interested in learning from my experience as a medical doctor. In 2010, he shared his vision for a new healing center in the Iquitos area. He invited a few of us to join him in this project, and eventually in 2011, Canadian artist/healer Cvita Mamic, Ricardo, and I became business partners. We founded the traditional healing center Nihue Rao (pronounced knee-way rao, rhymes with ow) Centro Espiritual. With the help of a wonderful team of individuals, we realized Ricardo's vision.

At Nihue Rao, as we call it, I began traditional apprenticeship under maestro Ricardo. Ricardo is a Shipibo shaman. The Shipibos are an indigenous people native to the Ucayali River basin in the Peruvian Upper Amazon. They have maintained much of their pre-Columbian culture, including their language and their mystical tradition of plant medicine.

Like many others, Ricardo had become a shaman after finding his own healing. After a difficult childhood and years of depression, in his late twenties, he turned to his own ancestral culture for help. By his own account, traditional Shipibo medicine and ayahuasca shamanism saved his life. The plants saved him from despair and helped him to build a new life, and he committed himself to working with the plants that healed him. He is a serious shaman and a youthful spirit.

For years, I worked alongside Ricardo in ayahuasca ceremony. These ceremonies were my classroom in the continued Fellowship of the River. Just as surgery is ultimately learned in the operating room, shamanism is learned in ceremony. At Nihue Rao, I gained valuable experience with a wide variety of cases.

During those years, I witnessed hundreds of Westerners, primarily from North America and Europe, benefit from traditional treatment with shamanic plant medicine, the course of their lives altered by powerful visions and shifted perceptions. In the chapters to follow, I will share the healing stories of Russ, Colleen, Nathan, and many others, in order to demonstrate how shamanic plant medicine and related spiritual techniques can help to heal many modern maladies and diseases—from post-traumatic stress disorder (PTSD) to chronic cough to Crohn's disease to anxiety and depression to a number of other psychosomatic conditions.

In the United States, as a physician, I have watched people spend years in frustration seeking treatment for these very same problems and related ailments. Despite spending thousands of dollars and consulting an army of specialists, many do not get to the root of their problem. Too often, the Western medical approach fails to address the emotional and spiritual dimensions of these chronic diseases and related illnesses, seeing them only as physical conditions. Shamanic plant medicine heals by going deeper into the emotional and spiritual realms; like other forms of spiritual healing, it works by altering our consciousness. As suggested by author Stephen Buhner, the mind is opened beyond the illusory limits of its current operating software.[1] The mind is opened to the heart and to the energies that disturb our emotional being.

Traditional medical philosophies like shamanism describe the presence of an "emotional body," through which we experience emotion and feeling. Modern science has also encountered this emotional body and is now able to describe its anatomy, a complex network that connects our psychology, our nervous system, our endocrine system, and our immune system. Emotional trauma and "spiritual wounds" impair this network and, in turn, compromise health.

The shamans have long known that when the emotional body is sick, the physical body cannot get well. Shamanic plant medicine gives us access to the mystical realms of the spirit, where we can find and heal these deeper wounds and release emotional burdens. Thus, emotional health returns and along with it our innate ability to heal mind and body.

After working with Ricardo for five years, I completed my initial shamanic training and became a beginner *ayahuasquero,* meaning that I could now conduct my own ayahuasca ceremonies and heal with shamanic song. I continued to work and practice at Nihue Rao until late 2016. As of this writing, the fellowship is complete, and I will be moving into some new ventures, although keeping my strong ties to the Amazonian community.

As with any medical fellowship, there is always much more to learn and practice, and I am most certainly still learning, but I also feel that it is time to share.

In chronic diseases in which the emotional body is ill, lasting healing will not be achieved until we address the needs of the heart and soul. One of the most profound ways I have found to achieve this is in ayahuasca ceremony within the context of the responsible practice of Traditional Amazonian Plant Medicine (TAPM).

The Fellowship of the River reintroduced me to the art of medicine, the value of spiritual healing, and inspired a further calling. I want to help build a bridge between the worlds of modern medical science and the mystical realms of traditional shamanism.

In the pages that follow, I will describe my own mysterious experiences in shamanism and I will share accounts of remarkable spiritual healings. As a doctor, I will attempt to weave modern clinical research into these mystical personal stories, referring to and reviewing relevant medical research from fields like psychedelic medicine, mind-body medicine, and epigenetics in the hopes of illuminating a broader medical paradigm.

The Fellowship of the River is a story, a series of stories really, about what nature's magic continues to teach us. Let's take a trip to the Amazon, and I'll show you what I mean.

# CHAPTER 2

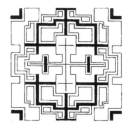

# The Plant Speaks

## "If you help me, I will help you"

A recognition of the spiritual essences inherent in nature is basic to the worldview of indigenous people, as it was for our ancestors in preindustrial societies.

—Ralph Metzner, PhD, *Sacred Vine of Spirits: Ayahuasca*

Keyvan and I began our fellowship with a flight to Iquitos, Peru. To be honest, I was scared to drink ayahuasca. I had heard that the experience could be extremely intense. Keyvan had told me not to worry. This would be his second round with ayahuasca, and he assured me that I would be all right, that she—*la Madre Ayahuasca*—would be a familiar friend, a guiding spirit.

Keyvan and I had first become friends during a field biology course in college. He is Persian-American, having moved to Los Angeles from Iran as a child, and often goes by the nickname Kave. He graduated college a year ahead of me, and we lost track of each other for a while. It turns out that he had gone on to several adventures, among them a Che Guevara–style sojourn across South America. After circling down and around Brazil, Uruguay, Argentina, and Bolivia, he had ended up alone in Iquitos, Peru. There, sometime in the late 1990s, he first met *la madrecita* Ayahuasca, Mother Ayahuasca, "the vine of the spirit."

Then in 2003, after completing my internship year back in my home state of Arizona, I ended up once again training with Keyvan at the UCLA Family Medicine program in Los Angeles. After our residency training we planned our initial trip to Peru, our "Fellowship of the River."

Keyvan was looking to complete the last leg of his loop through South America by heading down the Amazon River by boat from Iquitos to the north coast of Brazil. I also wanted to travel to Iquitos. After transformative experiences with peyote in Arizona, I was very curious to try the South American ayahuasca. I had read books like Jeremy Narby's *The Cosmic Serpent* and Rick Strassman's *DMT: The Spirit Molecule* and knew of ayahuasca's ability to induce profound and sometime life-changing visions, and that it is utilized in ceremonial healing throughout the Amazon rainforest. Thoughts of ayahuasca and its possibilities for teaching me and helping me personally had been swimming around in my head for some time, and the moment had finally arrived for me to experience it firsthand.

When Westerners say ayahuasca, what they are referring to is a tea made from ayahuasca vine (*Banisteriopsis caapi*) and other potent psychotropic plants native to the Amazon basin. Taken alone, the ayahuasca vine does not induce a psychedelic experience, but mixed into a tea with these other plants, it can induce powerful visions. In the Amazonian Shipibo tradition, which is the tradition into which I would later be initiated, ayahuasca is considered to be a healing spirit of nature, accessed by imbibing the ayahuasca tea in sacred ceremony. What happens in ayahuasca ceremony is that we connect to a spiritual intelligence beyond our ordinary comprehension. Most often people report contact with a form of plant consciousness. They call it the spirit of *la Madre* Ayahuasca. In this tradition, ayahuasca is regarded as feminine, a Mother Nature spirit of the forest. Through her, Mother Ayahuasca, we can access the healing wisdom of her plant spirit colleagues.

The word *ayahuasca* itself is taken from the Quechua language. *Aya* means death or spirit and *huasca* means vine, the spirit vine. This traditional medicine also has many other names among the diverse indigenous cultures of the extensive Amazonian region (*yagé, hoasca, caapi,* etc.).

Ayahuasca has become more and more widely known as a spiritual tool, and increasing numbers of people are flocking to the Amazon rainforest from all over the globe, seeking experiences with *la medicina,* participating in what is known as "ayahuasca tourism." Just as Keyvan and I did, they head to places like Iquitos, Peru, looking for an experience with Amazonian shamans, with the *ayahuasqueros* and the *ayahuasqueras.* There were other *gringos* on the flight from Lima to Iquitos. I imagine some of them were also seeking ayahuasca. Others were just travelling to the Amazon rainforest to tour its immense beauty.

Iquitos is a jungle-locked port city on the Amazon River. That is to say there are no roads linking Iquitos to the rest of Peru. You must arrive by air or by river. As you fly in, you can see the muddy brown Amazon winding through an ocean of emerald-green forest that extends as far as the eye can see. It is, as they say, deep in the jungle. Arriving at the small airport and stepping out of the plane, you are immediately greeted by the warm, musty air of the rainforest. That day, it was not too hot, a bit cloudy without rain.

After we got our luggage, we stepped outside to the "ground transportation" area. We had prearranged transportation from the airport to the ayahuasca healing center, and Marco Antonio the mototaxi driver had been waiting for us. He speaks some English and found us through the hustle and bustle of pushy *taxistas.* The mototaxi, part-motorcycle/part-rickshaw, cousin of the Asian *tuk tuk,* is the primary form of transportation in the busy city of Iquitos. Marco Antonio is a local and has been taking *pasajeros* ("passengers" on the journey, i.e., the participants in ayahuasca rituals) out to the ayahuasca centers for years. He is a kindred spirit who understands the concerns of Western seekers. Nowadays he continues to work with Nihue Rao. Just as he did that day, he always wears a bandana over his scalp and he always drives like a madman.

We let him know that we needed to get out to the center quickly, but he assured us that there was time to shoot through the city. The population of Iquitos is well into the hundreds of thousands and its streets are disorganized and chaotic. This is a bit overwhelming to the foreigner, but to the local, driving in Iquitos is considered fun. Marco Antonio raced us right through the open-air Belén market, honking his way through the crowded alleys as we passed countless stands selling everything from Tupperware to bushmeat.

Then we headed out of town to our destination, a traditional Shipibo healing center. Once you leave the city, things open up, the air gets cleaner, and you enter my favorite part of Iquitos, the jungle. After about 14 km on the main road out to Nauta, we turned on a dirt road north into the forest.

There were no longer many people around, and after a kilometer or so of sandy terrain we arrived at the guarded entrance to the healing center and lodge. They opened the gate and gave Marco Antonio the green light to barrel down a rickety Indiana Jones–style wooden bridge that took us right into the heart of the center. After a wild and bumpy ride filled with eruptions of nervous laughter, we made it.

What we found when we arrived was a large jungle compound with well-constructed wooden buildings organized around a large ceremonial space called a maloka. The maloka was known as the *Rao Shobo*, the medicine house in Shipibo.

There were showers and toilets and even a pool. The rustic thatched buildings were set in the forest ,and beyond them were multiple trails heading into the wilderness.

We settled into our assigned guestroom in the *casa grande*, a no frills, two-story wooden building that housed multiple guests. The rooms were spartan and mosquito-proof. We were oriented to the center primarily by the center's manager. She was friendly and generous with her knowledge.

We cruised around, got a feel for the place, and got to know our fellow *pasajeros*. There was a local man named Wilder cooking ayahuasca over an open fire. He was wearing a Phoenix Suns hat. I told him that I was from Phoenix. He smiled. For him it was just a hat.

I was interested to learn about how the ayahuasca was prepared. In Peru, ayahuasca tea is commonly prepared by boiling the shredded stalk of the woody vine with the leaves of the tryptamine-rich chacruna bush (*Psychotria viridis*). Chacruna is rich in dimethyltryptamine (DMT), the powerful hallucinogen responsible for inducing ayahuasca visions. There are a number of other ways to prepare ayahuasca tea, sometimes involving different tryptamine sources and/or the addition of other plants.

That first day we started our preparation by adopting a traditional Shipibo diet, referred to by some as a *vegetalista* diet. The vegetalista diet can vary considerably, depending on the prescribing shaman. At this center, we began with a plant-derived vomitive (which is exactly what it sounds like). Ours was a watery soup made from azucena (*Liliam spp*) and ojé (*Ficus insipida*). We were told that the plant-induced purge would cleanse us and prepare our stomachs for the ayahuasca. Let's just say it did the job.

We then started *la dieta:* no salt, no sugar, no red meat, no pork, no dairy, no oily food, no spicy food, no alcohol or drugs, and no sex. This was continued for the entirety of our five-day stay. Our meals consisted primarily of fish and plantains and a few other bland, starchy foods. The Shipibos believe that this cleansing diet is crucial to deeper healing with the plants, allowing for a stronger connection with the plant teachers. Per the tradition, the plants themselves have requested these dietary restrictions and have communicated this directly to the shamans through dreams and ayahuasca visions.

The following night we entered our first ceremony. I remember it vividly. I was anxious and scared as I entered the dimly lit maloka and took a spot on an available mat. This particular maloka or medicine house was a large jungle roundhouse big enough for about 25 people or so. Looking up, in the candlelight, I could appreciate its traditional Amazonian architecture. Natural wood beams formed a high conical ceiling, which was supported by a large central post. With its high ceiling, the maloka was like a thatched-roof cathedral. It had a natural dirt floor, covered in elegantly woven mats of some kind of natural fiber. These mats were smooth, soft, and intricate, like a snake's skin.

At the center of the space however the floor was left bare, exposed earth. In the ample space above us, there would be plenty of room for soaring thoughts and visions.

It was just after 8 p.m. I watched in the candlelight as others were called up to sit in front of the shaman and receive ayahuasca. One by one, we were given our dose of the tea, a small cup of murky liquid not entirely welcomed by the gut. Fortunately, my first dose of aya-huasca went down fairly easily, although, as I would later learn, this would not always be the case.

I headed back to my place with the peculiar taste of the thick jungle fluid lingering in my mouth. Waiting for the effect, I sat back on my thin mat and lit a mapacho cigarette, rolled from local Ama-zonian black tobacco (*Nicotiana rustica*). My new friends at the heal-ing center had told me that this would help clear the taste from my mouth. It did help, and so I puffed my mapacho, without inhaling as advised, and I sat back against the sturdy wooden wall supporting the sacred space.

Once all of the guests had been served their ayahuasca, the sha-mans served themselves, doing their best to savor their precious brew. Before the shamans drank, they sang into their ayahuasca. These early songs were more of a shush-shushing whistle, a rhythmic enchant-ment. In Spanish this is described as *soplando la ayahuasca*, "blowing" into it to infuse it with their intentions for the ceremonial healing. These *soplos* are a modest form of icaro, the mystical healing chant of the ayahuasca shamans.

According to the Shipibo, icaros are taught to the shamans by the plants themselves. Each *ayahuasquero* has his or her own icaros learned by dieting with master plants, the plants that teach us and guide us spiritually. The melody is directed by the plants, and the words are sung in Shipibo to address what is seen in the visions. Later in the night, as the ayahuasca took effect, we would hear the *ayahuasqueros* sing full-throated icaros, plant spirits singing through the voices of shamanic healers, with mystical intonation and vibra-tion. These icaros would guide our journeys into the world of the ayahuasca and its visions.

There were probably a dozen foreigners, both men and women, in ceremony that night, surrounded by the vibrant rain-forest night. Somewhere in the distance, the guards turned off the power and the rumbling gasoline generator rocked, rolled, and then purred to a halt.

We were in the jungle, la selva. As the lone candle was blown out, the darkness enveloped us, and the air began to fill with jungle song, the chirping, the buzzing, the croaking, and the whistling that watch over the jungle night. My eyes surrendered to the darkness, and I explored my mind and body for signs of "*la mareación*," the effects of the ayahuasca (*marear* in Spanish means to make sick, nauseous, dizzy, or confused). After about thirty minutes or so, I began to feel wavelike energies flowing from my head and throughout my body. I felt an expansion in my mind and in my chest, a disturbance in my vision. My breathing seemed to slow. My thoughts passed into feelings that pulsed through me, through my guts, and beyond my body. Before long, a strange heaviness overwhelmed me and I lay down.

At some point, I could see colors illuminating the dark. As the doors of perception began to open to a stranger dimension, the shamans broke the dark silence with their song, quietly at first, and then more fully. The ceremony increased in intensity as two or three of them sang together. I had never heard anything quite like that chanting, its impact no doubt amplified under the influence of the ayahuasca. The songs and their vibrations appeared to grip the energies of the visions, energies which seemed to flow right into and through me. I thought I heard someone vomit, but it did not disturb me.

The icaros filled the maloka and merged rhythmically with the sounds of the forest night. They filled my senses. It felt as if I were connecting to a new realm of consciousness, the world of the plants, so alien and yet so familiar.

As the songs continued, rhythmic, mystical, foreign, and beautiful, things got deeper and stranger. The chants felt like they were pulsing right through my soul, the icaros inspiring visions of geometric patterns and jungle scenery, like an intense dream. In the midst of all of the visions, I did not feel inebriated. My mind was clear. I knew I was in the maloka and I also knew that I was under the influence of the ayahuasca . . . and . . . it was also clear to me that I was being visited by a spiritual entity.

There were reverberating sounds and strobe-like visual ripples. A female spirit came to greet me amidst rapidly changing images of rainforest scenery and phantasmagoric bats and growling faces. This spirit was both frightening and beautiful, friendly and seductive, sweet and severe. Her face changed rapidly, portraying varied countenances that were all at once terrifying, loving, inspiring, and sexy. Her hair and body were composed of wildly flowing vines, covered in leaves, with green and orange tones. Dancing light surrounded her.

I was completely mesmerized by her. She reached her hand down to me and invited me to join her. She could see that I was a bit lonely and she flirted with me as she pulled me into the dream and took me on a journey. We left the maloka, and we left the night. She gently guided me on a stroll to a lakeside beach and we stepped into the sunshine. There was a translucent haze in some moments; other moments were illuminated from below. There was a very clear landscape, sunlight glimmering off the lake, the rich green forest surrounding us, and a lovely blue sky. We found a peaceful place to lie down, grassy and sandy, and there we were. I spent the afternoon with her, lying on the beach, enjoying her lovely company.

I knew who she was. *La Madre* Ayahuasca. I could not be sure, but I was sure. I had heard about her—spirit of nature, a plant spirit, a living extension of earth and divine light. She drew me into a magical realm that felt so real, that seemed to be in continuum with my consciousness.

After our very pleasant and otherworldly afternoon, in a place beyond time, she guided me back into the night, to my spot in the maloka. She looked at me one last time, intensely, and left me with these parting words, "If you help me, I will help you." It was as if she blew them straight into my consciousness where they just reverberated, unforgettable.

If you help me, I will help you.

After a while, I could feel the most intense effects wearing off. I rolled to one side to check on my friend Keyvan. "How are you?" I whispered.

"This is gnarly, y *tu loco*?" he said.

"Definitely gnarly," I replied, the visuals still fading.

The ceremony quieted and seemed to move into a second phase. Ricardo the assistant shaman broke the silence and asked the group, "*Alguien quiere más ayahuasca*?" In his playful tone, the offer seemed a bit mischievous. He was offering a second round. I did not feel sick, I felt generally well, but after having experienced what seemed to be an eternity of near-catatonic visual experience, I thought I would pass. Out of nowhere, an amazingly composed Keyvan sat up and called out, "*Yo sí*." Okay, I thought, here we go again. We took the second dose.

The second dose took me on more of a profound internal journey. Peacefully, I lay there in the darkness and reviewed my life and my perceived problems. Again, some unknown amount of time passed in this exploration, fueled and guided by the mysterious icaros of the shamans.

As the effect calmed a bit, I withdrew from my introspection. I wondered where she had gone, the beautiful spirit of ayahuasca. Just as I thought to look for her again, I glimpsed her slipping out the door of the maloka . . . I had just missed her. Whether I saw her or not, I knew she was with me.

Still feeling the effect in my head and body, I was then visited in the dark by the giggling shaman Ricardo Amaringo. In the dark I was convinced that he was somebody else. I thought for sure he was the ayahuasca cook I had met earlier in the day, the one with the Phoenix Suns hat. I asked him, "*Quién eres*?" Who are you?

He could see that I was a bit lost in the effect, and rather than stirring my mind further with a verbal response, he giggled and observed, tuning in to my state. Trying to seem more together, I then said, "I know who you are." He simply laughed again and continued his observations, sitting close in the pitch darkness. At the prescribed moment, he opened with his song. His icaro blasted me with a brilliant light that revved up the ayahuasca throughout my entire body. I could feel every cell in my body buzzing with life. At some point, his leg had brushed against mine. I felt smooth snakeskin and the muscular girth of a large boa constrictor. A vision of snakeskin patterns flashed across my mind.

Afterwards, I thanked him for his song, amazed by the brilliant light it generated in my visions. Ricardo asked me about my experience. In particular, I mentioned that I felt his leg become a snake. He laughed and whispered across the darkness, "That's the ayahuasca." He blew some mapacho smoke on me from his pipe and then quietly moved on to the next person.

Eventually the ceremony wound down once more. After a final chant, it was announced that the ceremony was closed, and that we could break our silence and talk amongst ourselves. The post-ceremonial conversation confirmed that we had just been through an incredible experience. Some of the others went back to their room to rest; I stayed in the maloka.

I was in awe. I did not sleep a wink that night, and yet I greeted the sunrise feeling totally clear and refreshed.

*If you help me, I will help you.* The words lingered in my mind.

# CHAPTER 3

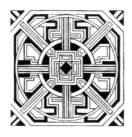

# The Wounded Healer

bless the thing
that broke you down
and cracked you
open
because the world
needs you open

—Rebecca Campbell

People often ask me how I, a medical doctor from the United States, ended up in Peru, communicating with plant spirits. Well, the answer is that I have always been interested in "alternative" and integrative medicine. I suppose it's somewhat unusual for a Western-trained MD to be quite so interested in other forms of healing, but I was never really on a standard medical path.

I was raised in a spiritually oriented Colombian-American family. I grew up hearing stories about miraculous healings in South America and other parts of the world. As a child of immigrants, I was always curious about different cultural perspectives.

My father was a medical doctor. After working in general practice in Colombia, he decided to train in psychiatry in the United

States. When my older brother was just a baby, the family moved to Missouri and then to Kansas, where my younger brother and I were born. Once my father completed his psychiatry residency, he found work in Phoenix, Arizona, where I spent my formative years.

From an early age, I thought about becoming a medical doctor like my father, but I was also interested in other systems of medicine. In Arizona, I encountered Native American traditional medicine, and later in California, I was exposed to Traditional Chinese Medicine and West African spiritual healing. That early exposure to various healing traditions kept me open to and curious about the dimensions of health that are often overlooked by Western medicine.

I was premed in college but by the time I graduated in 1996, I had changed my mind. I wasn't sure that I fit into the premed culture and decided to look for something further off the beaten path. I briefly explored a career as a field biologist, but before long, I drifted back to healthcare. For about nine months or so, I worked as a treatment advocate for Latino AIDS patients in Los Angeles. Through this work I was exposed to acupuncture, energy healing, and a few other "alternative" therapies. In L.A., I was also exposed to a number of religious and spiritual practices, ranging from Japanese Zen meditation to Afro-Cuban Santeria.

In 1998 I followed my then-girlfriend to San Diego. She helped me find work at a facility that cared for emotionally disturbed teens. Several months later I got a job in health education at the UCSD Student Healthcare Clinic (right across the way from the UCSD medical school). While working there, I took an introductory course at the Pacific College of Oriental Medicine (PCOM), and for some time considered studying acupuncture and herbal medicine.

My father, a dedicated physician, had been concerned about my wanderings. He saw that I was interested in the growing integrative and "alternative" medicine movement and suggested to me that in his opinion the best way to change the system was from *within*. He encouraged me to become a medical doctor so that I might one day do something more integrative. Eventually, I followed his advice.

During my application process for medical school, I interviewed at the UCSD School of Medicine (SOM). It was while touring the campus that I ran into my college friend Keyvan. I had not seen him for a few years. It was good to see him and we caught up briefly. Keyvan had started medical school there the year before. As we wrapped up our conversation, he was compelled to warn me about the program. He described the environment as rather cold, and was concerned that it would be hard on me and my unconventional spirit. His first year had been rough and he was considering taking some time off.

I ended up getting into UCSD. Despite Keyvan's warning, I entered medical school there in the fall of 1999. I am very grateful to the UCSD SOM, and I am very proud to be a doctor. Being an MD has opened many doors in my life, and my work as a medical doctor has been, on many occasions, very rewarding. But it's not all flowers, as they say. I had a hard time in medical school and I learned some tough lessons about mental suffering and soul sickness. This suffering is what drove me to seek healing from the plants. Ironically, medical school was the road that brought me to the Fellowship of the River.

A 2016 study estimated that almost one third of US medical students are depressed.[1] I was one of those depressed students. As I look back on that period, I remember what Ricardo the shaman says about depression. He believes that most depression is caused by anger.

I was angry in medical school, angry about entering a medical culture that didn't seem to care enough about us, the future of medicine. Rather than feeling supported, I think many of us were afraid. Exposing a problem was a threat to your professional future. I remember reviewing a dip in my academic performance with the administration. I had failed a class during my second year.

"Maybe you should tell me what happened. Unless you can make us understand what was going on, I'm going to have to let the residencies know about your depressive tendencies, we'll have to put something in your file," the woman said to me behind closed doors.

I didn't care to share anything about myself with her. Maybe I was too proud, but I didn't feel genuine concern in her tone. "I think you should put down whatever you feel is right," I replied.

I was angry about having to tolerate disrespectful behavior from those who would take advantage of this culture of fear. Perhaps it was just a few bad apples, but I was tired of professors and teachers interested in publicly and privately humiliating us. People, who in my opinion, looked frustrated and unhappy themselves. My father and his friends loved their work, but maybe the culture of medicine was changing, or maybe I was just getting to know a less-satisfied group of doctors. (In 2015, Medscape Physician Lifestyle reported that 46 percent of US medical doctors report burnout, up from 40 percent in 2013.[2])

I was angry about not knowing if all the hard work was worth it. In my frustration, I turned this anger on myself. Inside my mind, I became hypercritical and increasingly insecure. I was trapped in my thoughts, losing touch with the world around me. I felt ashamed for feeling so lost and didn't know what to do. So I went to the student health center and complained about my breathing, and, as you'll recall, was diagnosed with "medical school syndrome."

Later, in the third and fourth years, working with patients provided me with a sense of purpose and gave me the motivation to tolerate the disturbing culture. But the first two years, the indoctrination, depressed me. Despite a positive group of friends to support me through the process, my world became darker and darker. I tried to stay connected to the things that nourished me, natural settings and natural people, but it was too much to maintain, and I cracked.

I tried to stuff down my negative feelings, my anger, my insecurity, my sadness, but it didn't help. I didn't want to feel anymore. I tried to close myself off from my feelings. Unfortunately, in doing this, I lost my connection to faith.

Why, for some, is training to become a doctor so depressing? Why does work as a doctor lead to so much burnout?

Well, I think it's because our materialist culture has created a system that is too hard on us, too hard on our hearts. Our culture and our healthcare system are increasingly managed by corporate values. We are losing touch with human values. In our current healthcare system, too often, material gain takes priority over the health and happiness of both patients and practitioners. We are too busy to make time for how we feel.

A culture that denies its natural empathy is dehumanized. The mind cannot deny the heart, not for long. The body cannot sustain this. This denial breaks the body down. Humans cannot deny their humanity, not for long.

As a culture, we are beginning to remember this. In order to be healthy and whole, we must be in touch with ourselves, our communities, and our environment. African traditional healer and scholar Dr. Malidoma Somé has diagnosed Western society as being disconnected from three basic human necessities: nature, community, and ritual (which provides a channel to access spirit).

I felt *connected* before medical school, connected to myself, to nature, community, and spirit. Somewhere in those first two years, I lost this connection. In turn, my faith faded away, and I became depressed.

In traditional medicine, in cultures all over the world, the personal well-being of the healer is prioritized. This is true even if the training itself is potentially traumatizing. Training to become a traditional Shipibo shaman is difficult and rigorous. In the lineage with which I am familiar (under maestro Ricardo Amaringo), the official preparation involves a one-year *vegetalista* diet in isolation in the forest, without social influences, without alcohol/drugs, sex, salt, sugar, spices, fats, dairy, pork, or red meat. In one very strict format, the trainees (dieters) eat only certain types of grilled fish and plantains, with some water, maybe some plantain juice, and that's it. They speak only minimally. People are assigned to care for these trainees as they become malnourished and weak. They sacrifice themselves and they are broken down. Their egos and public personas fade away, making room for spirit to come forward.

Despite the obvious difficulties, throughout the process they are encouraged to open their minds and stay connected to their hearts. At Nihue Rao, I have seen several individuals complete the strict one-year diet. They suffer, but ultimately, they are fortified. As Ricardo says, their bodies are weak but their minds and spirits become stronger.

Once their diets are closed, they begin to eat and live normally, and in a month or two, their weakened bodies recover. Typically, the dieters (*dieteros*) finish better than when they started, more whole in mind, body, and spirit.

I went through a form of this training process, which I will describe later. My *vegetalista* diets certainly left me healthier than when I started.

I cannot say the same for my allopathic medical training. I was traumatized and broken down, but there was no plan to build me back up. This is the rat-race culture, which overextends itself without a plan for recovery. Health and vitality are overlooked for the promise of material success.

In medical school, I learned many important and fascinating things, and I also learned what it is to be disconnected from my heart. Like many others, I became trapped in my mind, trapped in negative thinking, self-doubt, and self-criticism.

Looking back, I can now see that this depression was something that I had to go through. I was a frustrated healer going through a necessary initiation, and although I am grateful *now*, it was hard back *then*.

During those years, when I would go back to visit Arizona, my family would see me down and moping around. This was out of character for me. It was difficult to explain myself. Medical school was supposed to be a grand opportunity, but it didn't seem so grand to me. I think my father's medical school experience in Colombia was quite different. In his culture, there was more respect for human emotion and spirituality. While at home, I would try to rest and keep to myself, but eventually I would invariably start complaining about my choice to study medicine. I told my family that the school was making me sick, that the faculty wanted me to suck up to people that I did not respect, and that the experience was too often heartless.

Then I would head back to school. I continued to feel worse, and I knew I needed help. One thing that really did help me was going to a sweat lodge outside of San Diego, with an Apache shaman, Maria.

She had been guest lecturing at a medical anthropology course on campus. I resonated with her native perspective; it felt encouraging and healing.

My family was increasingly concerned, especially my father. Up to that point, I had not personally known him as a healer. Psychiatry is a discreet profession and he didn't bring his work home very much. But then one day, something shifted.

I was visiting my parents in Arizona again. He was sitting at his computer just passing the time. He saw me looking kind of screwed up and he stopped me. He asked me why I was so sad, and for some reason I froze. Something about his energy, the tone of his voice, the way he looked at me, brought all of my emotions to the surface. My father became the healer. His presence opened something inside of me and I broke into tears, releasing much of the grief I had been carrying. I hadn't cried in a very long time.

I shared my feelings with him and later with my mother. They were concerned and supportive. This was toward the end of the second year and I still had plenty of marching to do. He suggested that I try an antidepressant medication for a while. Knowing my mind, he was quite certain that citalopram, an SSRI (selective serotonin reuptake inhibitor), would help. I was embarrassed to try it, but I really needed relief (I would later discover that a number of my fellow students were also being treated with antidepressants).

I took citalopram for about six weeks. It did help me. My negative thoughts were still around but they were not so consuming. I was not so disconnected from the outside world. I could appreciate a nice day in a way that I had forgotten about. I had a better sense of myself, and it was easier to smile.

I was happy with the treatment, but did notice a few strange side effects. I noticed a strange aura at the periphery of my vision. This reminded me of something that I had experienced with psilocybin mushrooms, which I had experimented with a handful of times. I also felt tension in my jaw, similar to what I felt once when I tried Ecstasy, a popular mood-altering psychedelic created from 3,4-methylenedioxy-methamphetamine (MDMA).

The antidepressants helped, but I wanted to be healed, and after six weeks, I decided to stop. Not because of side effects, but because it just did not feel right for me. (One should always talk with a doctor before stopping antidepressants. Some of these medications require a weaning-off period.) I don't remember if I mentioned anything to my dad.

I was interested in finding a more natural remedy. A spiritual approach would be the key. I discovered this on the peyote way.

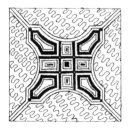

# CHAPTER 4

# Peyote Way

Peyote is a sacrament for all—no one church, race, or government can "own" it.

—Reverend Immanuel Trujillo, Peyote Way Church of God

I was still in medical school when I had my first experience with spiritual plant medicine. I entered peyote ceremony at the Peyote Way Church of God in Arizona. Peyote has been used as a sacrament at this legally recognized church since its establishment in the late 1970s, where it is experienced in a ceremony known as the Spirit Walk. My first Spirit Walk gave me the strength to complete my medical training.

In medical school, as you've seen, I had become trapped in my mind—in spiraling negative thoughts. I was cut off from my heart and feelings, disconnected. In just one night, peyote helped me to reconnect. It quieted and opened my mind, helping me to reconnect to everything that was most important to me. Of course I had more work to do, but peyote got me back on track.

Growing up in Arizona, I had heard a few things about peyote cactus. I knew that it was strongly psychoactive and that it was used as a traditional medicine in certain Native American traditions. In college, I had read about peyote (*mescalito*) in Carlos Castaneda's book *The Teachings of Don Juan*. This book was my first exposure to the idea of working with a plant spirit as an ally. This idea appealed to me.

Peyote (*Lophophora williamsii*) is a small, spineless, slow-growing cactus native to Mexico and parts of the Southwestern United States. It contains, among other things, the psychedelic alkaloid mescaline, which is concentrated most strongly at the top of the little plant. Without harming the plant, the top section of the cactus can be carefully harvested as what's called a "peyote button" for ceremonial use. These buttons can be eaten fresh or dried and can be made into powder or tea. Archaeologic evidence indicates that peyote has been used in ceremony in North America for over 5000 years.[1,2]

Like ayahuasca, peyote is central to a number of diverse traditions, in Mexico and the United States. Today, the most widely practiced peyote tradition in the United States is that of the Native American Church (NAC). Despite the fact that some consider peyote a "drug," the US Supreme Court has officially recognized the NAC's religious right to work with peyote as a sacrament. (This precedent has led to further legal statutes that protect the sacramental use of peyote at places like the Peyote Way Church of God.)

I was interested in trying peyote for my depression. Although I had benefitted from the antidepressant, I was interested in a deeper treatment, something that went beyond daily modulation of my brain chemistry. I was interested in finding something more natural. I was, however, apprehensive about taking peyote, having heard that it was a "strong" psychedelic. I had had only minimal experience with psychedelic mushrooms and Ecstasy and was generally fearful of getting more involved. I was also aware of the stigma around "hallucinogens," that they are dangerous substances that can make you flip your lid (for good). Antidepressants have their own stigma too, that they are for the weak that can't handle life. But they also have the backing of a massive pharmaceutical industry with generous research budgets, government approval, physician endorsement, and favorable press. Not so for peyote.

Somehow I managed to wrap my head around the idea and, stigma or not, I decided to give peyote a try.

During my third year in medical school I found an opportunity to participate in peyote ceremony. I had been learning about a renaissance in psychedelic research from my good friend and classmate Barack. He had entered medical school with the intention of doing research on altered states of consciousness, in particular on those induced by meditation and psychedelics. This seemed crazy, particularly at our generally conservative institution, but times are changing and he pulled it off.

# History of Psychedelic Medicine

Barack directed me to the astonishing world of psychedelic research. Since their scientific discovery in the 1940s, psychedelics like LSD and mescaline had been subject to clinical investigation. They were studied for decades for their potential as medications. During this time, the field of psychopharmacology—the study of pharmaceutical effects on mood, sensation, thinking, and behavior—came into being. Basically, everything we know about the brain's chemistry has come from psychopharmacological studies, and for thirty years, psychedelics were part of that effort.

Early psychedelic research started in 1943 with the accidental discovery of LSD by Swiss chemist Albert Hoffman. Subsequent research led to the chemical isolation of psilocybin from "magic" mushrooms traditionally utilized by Mazatec shamans in southern Mexico. Research on these psychedelic substances and others played a pivotal role in understanding the activity of neurotransmitters in the human brain.[3] Neurotransmitters like serotonin, for example, are molecular messengers that help nerve cells in the brain communicate with one another. Neurotransmitters are the current focus of modern psychopharmacology and most psychiatric pharmaceutical treatment.

After three decades of promising research, in the late 1960s, clinical research into psychedelic medicines was brought to an abrupt stop. By then LSD had developed its reputation as a party drug among the "hippies," it was being sold on the streets, and the establishment had become uncomfortable with its disruptive influence. By 1968, possession of most psychedelics had become illegal in the United States Clinical research was halted, despite promising evidence that substances like LSD and MDMA (Ecstasy/Molly) could be used in the treatment of addiction and deep psychological trauma.[4-7]

Early psychedelic research had advanced our understanding of the mood-altering serotonin (also known as 5-hydroxy*tryptamine* or 5-HT) system and its role in psychology. The serotonin system, the network of brain cells that relies most heavily on the neurotransmitter serotonin, is the target of some of the most widely prescribed antidepressants, including the SSRIs (once again, Selective Serotonin Reuptake Inhibitors), e.g., Prozac and the citalopram I was prescribed. Before talking to Barack, I had not realized that elements of the serotonin system are also one of the primary targets of psychedelic pharmaceuticals like LSD, psilocybin, and DMT.[4-7]

SSRI antidepressants and the psychedelics are biochemically connected. This connection underlies their mutual utility in the treatment of certain mental health problems. It also explains why the antidepressant citalopram made me feel like I was on a low dose of psilocybin mushrooms.

With the criminalizing of psychedelic substances, they were re-classified as Schedule I Narcotics. This is the Drug Enforcement Agency's (DEA) classification for substances alleged to have a high abuse potential, safety concerns, and no accepted medicinal use. This is a controversial classification, as it goes against evidence that indicates that at least some psychedelics do not meet Schedule I criteria.[5-11]

No prescriptions may be written for Schedule I substances; without DEA exemption, Schedule I substances are not available for therapeutic use or research. (States can however challenge this federal regulation, as they have in the case of medical marijuana.)

I suppose it's unsurprising that none of this history was covered in my medical school curriculum.

Official scientific research into the activity of these psychoactive substances began again in the 1990s. In 1991, Dr. Rick Strassman was the first investigator to gain permission from the DEA to re-open psychedelic research with his DMT study at the University of New Mexico.[12] Since that time, science and medicine have been taking a second look at psychedelics. The DEA has since granted further research exemptions allowing for a growing number of investigations and clinical trials in the United States. These studies and research abroad have shown great promise in the treatment of a number of mental health problems, including PTSD (post-traumatic stress disorder), addiction, anxiety, and depression.[5,6,13-15]

## Bona Fide Religious Use

As I learned more about the relationship between psychedelics and psychiatric medicine, I grew more comfortable with the idea of seeking healing from a mystical cactus. On a road trip across the Sonoran Desert from San Diego to Arizona, Barack convinced me to contact the Peyote Way Church of God in Klondyke. After some awkward email exchanges with the Church, in which they advised us not to come, and a trip that included 26 miles down a dirt road, Barack and I found ourselves in front of the church on a Sunday afternoon. Barack was on his relatively flexible research schedule. I on the other hand was supposed to be back to San Diego (about 600 miles away) the following morning to start my deadly serious Surgery Rotation.

The Reverend Anne Zapf had fielded our emails. She was the one who explained that peyote ceremony at the church requires proper planning and that our plans were too rushed, making a Spirit Walk highly unlikely. But that was okay with us. We figured we'd meet the folks at the church and visit for a few hours or so. That would still give us enough time to make it back for Monday morning lecture.

The church sits in desert ranching territory in southeastern Arizona, deep in the remote Aravaipa wilderness. Its property is just down the road from the Aravaipa Canyon Preserve, a lovely wooded oasis with a year-round stream. The area has been inhabited by native peoples for millennia, most recently by members of the Apache Nation. It is a beautiful location known traditionally for its clay pottery.

The main church is a converted house lovingly decorated with art produced by church founders the Reverend Immanuel Trujillo, the Reverend Anne Zapf, her husband Rabbi Matthew Kent, and their family. They are spiritualists and artists working in visual art and ceramics. Upon arrival, we encountered the informative and kind Rabbi Matthew, covered in white pottery dust, walking in our direction.

We explained to him that although we knew it was very unlikely, we were interested in experiencing the sacrament if at all possible. Despite my schedule, we were still hoping for a chance. He directed us to speak to his wife, Anne. We respectfully pleaded with her. She directed us to check out the library while she thought it over. Anne returned after an hour or so and was willing to offer us an opportunity. She explained what would be required.

In order to Spirit Walk, we would have to fast for 24 hours on the church property, beginning after dinner that night. Our Spirit Walk would not be until Monday. We would make our donation and spend the next day in reverent preparation exploring the church's 160 acres of desert wilderness. We would not be able to return to San Diego until Tuesday at the earliest. This meant I would not be able to show up to my surgery rotation until Wednesday, two days late. I was a bit unnerved, but I could not turn down this opportunity. I was determined to discover what peyote could offer. We agreed.

That afternoon, we helped to prepare the peyote buttons for our tea. Sitting around the kitchen table, Anne readied us for the experience, explaining the layout of the property and where we could go during our ceremony.

After dinner we hung out around the church house. That night I read through a copy of *The Little Prince* by Antoine de Saint-Exupéry, which I had found in the church library. At one point in the story a fox tells the little prince, "One sees clearly only with the heart. What is essential is invisible to the eyes."

The desert was very peaceful that night. The quiet helped calm my med student worries.

I called the medical school from the church on Monday morning and told them that I would be delayed for two days because my car had broken down in the Arizona desert. The conversation did not go very well. The rotation coordinator was not impressed or just didn't believe me. Voices were raised and then he threatened to make me repeat the twelve-week rotation. Another twelve weeks!!! Unbelievable, I thought—for missing the first two days of introductory lectures. My heart sank. It was already too late.

Then surprisingly enough, he sighed and changed his tone. He said he would need to talk to my faculty advisor about all of this . . . before deciding anything. That was music to my ears. My faculty advisor, Joyce, was definitely one of the angels that helped me through med school. I called and left a message with Joyce telling her about the problem with the car. I begged her to help me, I hung up, and then let it go. I was worried but I started to get the feeling that things were going to be all right.

The Spirit Walk involves first drinking a ceremonial dose of peyote tea at an outdoor site on church property and then remaining in nature for the Walk, ideally under the stars and alone. To paraphrase Reverend Immanuel, social contact pressures you to present your personality and your ego, both of which interfere with deeper spiritual contact. But it is permissible to Spirit Walk with others. Barack and I decided to go through the experience together. He was very experienced with psychedelics and I was a bit afraid. We agreed to respect each other's space and minimize conversation.

We spent the early part of the day cruising around the property to find a location. The church staff helped us to set up a comfortable campsite with a fire pit and lounge chairs. Late in the afternoon we met up with Anne to receive our mason jars full of peyote tea. We were each given a pint of strong tea to drink slowly over two hours (this is a much greater quantity of tea than what one drinks in ayahuasca ceremony). Drinking it slowly helps keep it down. Peyote can be quite nauseating. If you are not careful you can throw it all up before it is well absorbed.

Once you drink it, you are on the Spirit Walk, whether you're in a lounge chair or up on your feet. The experience can last until morning, with some continued effects lasting into the next day.

We headed to our campsite and got started in the early evening. At first it did not taste too bad, but as I worked my way down the jar, it got increasingly bitter. The last sips were revolting. My lips rebelled, involuntarily darting away from that relentless jar, but after a slow and steady struggle, I managed to get it all down and so did Barack.

Many things happened that night, of which I will mention only a few. The beginning was a bit rough for me. I was envious of Barack's calm. He appeared to be quietly meditating on the ground next to the fire. Not me. For some unknown period in purgatory, I was rolling back and forth on the lounge chair praying for my guts to settle down. Something definitely felt wrong. It all started to seem like a terrible mistake. I had foolishly wandered into a miserable night, and to make matters worse, I was probably going to have to repeat my surgery rotation. Rats!

There I was, suffering in my regret for what seemed like hours. Then at some magical moment everything shifted. My guts calmed a bit. I looked up. The night sky was beautiful. Dazzling stars were beaming down. The temperature felt comfortable. I felt comfortable. I sat up. I could sense something shifting in my mind. I felt a presence inside and also around me. It was peyote, "mescalito." I looked across the campfire to Barack.

"Mescalito is here," I reported.

He quietly nodded in agreement. We sat for some time at the fire and then decided to take a silent walk. The desert calm pierced my senses. A ringing in my ear was pulling my thoughts apart but it wasn't uncomfortable. We cruised along together for a while and then I walked on ahead. At some point, Barack had bent down on one knee to receive what appeared to be some kind of cosmic transmission. I kept walking down the perceivable trail, and the medicine seemed to peak. My vision became pixelated and I started to approach what looked like a horse in the distance. In my altered state, I began to consider the possibility that I was actually in the original *Clash of the Titans* movie approaching the winged Pegasus. It was in fact the church's mare, Molly. I got pretty close. At some point Barack stood up and started looking for me. Once he saw me, he caught up quickly. We spooked the horse and she bolted away.

Barack then asked me, "Do you smell that, what that horse just put out?"

Then I smelled it too, kind of a mix of urine and hay and something musky. Just then, her stallion boyfriend came stampeding out of the darkness, huffing and puffing, scaring us back. We had smelled her pheromones and so had he. It was startling and fantastic. We apologized and backed away. The situation dissipated.

A little later, we sat down on a gravelly hill. By then the effect had calmed, and for the most part my vision had cleared. Overall, I was feeling great, peaceful and overjoyed. One of the church's cats, a tabby, had wandered over to us, brushed past us, and then wandered off.

I just sat there feeling immense gratitude. My mind was quiet, no internal dialogue, none. I was not criticizing myself, I didn't feel insecure. My consciousness was filled by my senses and a sense of just being. Instead of being preoccupied, trying to figure out who I was, I was simply being myself . . . without commentary. In that state, with my mind so calm and quiet, I could finally feel compassion for myself. I realized that in general my life was moving in a positive direction. I felt connected to my heart and to the universe, my mind wide open, and I found hope. Faith was not just an abstract concept, but a tangible connection to a larger universe, the feeling of participating in all that is.

Then my thoughts were directed toward the ways I had hurt others in my reckless suffering, a girlfriend whose feelings I did not consider, things that I could have done better. The peyote had opened a space for me to contemplate without judgment and make plans to improve my behavior.

I had not thrown up during that ceremony, as is so common with peyote, but late in the night I let Barack know that I needed to make it back to the church house to use the bathroom. As we approached the front porch, we ran into Reverend Immanuel. It must have been three or four in the morning. He was standing out there looking out into the darkness. He was advanced in age, a veteran of World War II who had found his way back to his native roots in Arizona. After years as a NAC medicine man, he had started the Peyote Way Church with Matt and Anne. Living out there, he knew stillness. He was standing there in his bathrobe, with his long white hair and his unambiguous eyes. It was as if he were waiting for us there. He had been painting all night in his room. He was chewing a button and I could smell the peyote on his breath.

We talked for a while about medicine and desert dwelling. He was very kind that night.

The next day I bought a nice "Peyote Way" t-shirt to remind me of my experiences in the desert. Eventually we got back on the road to San Diego. I showed up to lectures on Wednesday, and no one even noticed. Two of our female classmates had gotten trapped in a hurricane in Cabo San Lucas for the whole week. News of their ordeal swept away any issue over my absence. It turned out to be no problem. (They also made it back safely.)

The Spirit Walk was well worth the risk. That night turned me around. After months and months of mental suffering, the peyote ceremony had not only quieted my mind and shown me what was possible, it had given me a chance to reset.

# CHAPTER 5

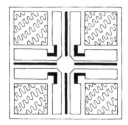

# Mind, Feeling, and Faith

I saw a soul in hell
For hell is the spirit prevented
From going on, it is time
Arrested in the nothingness
Between two states of being

—Laurens van der Post

Thanks to the peyote, I made it through the rest of medical school. The Spirit Walk had gotten me back on track with myself and given me a sense of connection and a sense of purpose. Sometime afterward, I decided to specialize in family medicine. This specialty appeared to provide the broadest educational and training opportunities, and a potential pathway toward a career in integrative medicine.

After medical school, I moved back to Phoenix for one year to complete my Family Medicine internship at St. Joseph's Hospital. Internship was a chance to utilize my hard-earned medical knowledge, and I enjoyed it. Western medicine has some blind spots, but as I know very well, it continues to save lives and help many, many people.

I had a positive experience at St. Joseph's but was eager to get back to California, and toward the end of that year, Keyvan called to let me know about an opening at the UCLA program. One of their residents had a military obligation and was about to be deployed to the Middle East. And so, in 2004, I moved back to balmy Los Angeles to complete my residency training.

The UCLA Family Medicine Residency was also a good experience. The faculty members were in general kind and open-minded. While there, I had the opportunity to further explore acupuncture and Traditional Chinese Medicine diagnosis at the UCLA Center for East-West Medicine. As a resident, I spent more and more time in the outpatient setting at the family medicine clinic. I gained experience with patients, the larger community and the healthcare system. I also returned to the Peyote Way Church several times, alone and with friends.

Meanwhile, my older brother Mario had also moved to the Los Angeles area. For some years, Mario had been working at Amnesty International championing human rights, connecting Angelinos to the global struggle against oppression. In his work at the Los Angeles office he met a wide variety of people, among them, Hollywood celebrities, political dissidents, and indigenous chiefs.

One evening Mario stopped by my apartment and asked me if I wanted to "go and hang out with some Bushmen from the Kalahari." Properly known as the San people of Southern Africa, the so-called "Bushmen" are said to be the descendants of the oldest culture on earth. I had first learned about them from the eighties movie *The Gods Must Be Crazy* (set in Botswana). I had also seen San people in *National Geographic* and in documentaries, living simply, deep in the wilderness. I remembered hearing their distinctive language with its varied tones and clicking sounds. Yes! I definitely wanted to hang out with the Bushmen.

A contingent of San people from Botswana and South Africa were touring to raise money and awareness for their land rights case in Botswana. They and their coalition of supporters were being hosted at Mario's friend's house in West Los Angeles. Mario had been invited to the gathering, and I was going along as his guest.

It was a clear, cool evening. Mario knew the way. Upon arrival, we entered through the side gate and joined the diverse group of twelve or so in the large backyard. They had some tents set up and a decent-sized fire going. We greeted everyone and mingled into the friendly atmosphere. I had my Peyote Way t-shirt on. It was blue-green with a stylized deer and peyote cactus printed on the front. I wandered around and came across their political leader, Roy Sesana, a native of the Kalahari Desert. After some brief conversation, he zeroed in on my t-shirt.

"I like your shirt," he said in his gravelly English. "Give it to me!"

The temperature was dropping and I told him I would have to give it to him later. I told him about the design, about the peyote and the American Southwest. This piqued his interest. After a few further questions, he asked me where he could get some of this peyote. I let him know that that would be difficult.

As the evening progressed, we became friends. (The next day I gave him the shirt. He kindly returned the favor and gave me an oryx tail flyswatter.)

At some point I took a seat around the fire with the others. As they have for tens of thousands of years, our new San friends began to tell stories. Many of them were born and raised in the bush or had at the very least lived in the bush for many years, hunting and gathering amongst rhinos and elephants. There were tales of hunting kudus on horseback, braving leopard attacks, and staring down lions.

One of the guests was a traditional San healer from South Africa. Dressed warmly for the California night, he stood up smiling, ready to poke fun at us. We welcomed the cultural exchange.

"Why do people get nightmares? Do you know, can any of you remember?" he said. "Does anyone know why people get nightmares?"

The crowd shouted various answers. He dismissed each one and swiped it away, "No! No! No! You've forgotten everything! You've forgotten everything! . . . Forget that question."

"Let me ask you this. Why does the Bushman always sleep like this?" he asked as he demonstrated.

"The Bushman always sleeps curled up on one side and rests his head on his cupped hand. As he rests his head on his hand, his hand is cupped to his ear. Why does the Bushman sleep like that?"

Again the crown fired away, "Oh, for the bugs," "yes, for the insects . . . ," "yeah!" and again he expressed his disappointment.

"No, no, no, no! You have forgotten everything."

Then he explained. In the bush, the Bushman sleeps like that so that he can rest more comfortably. The cupped hand amplifies vibrations and sounds from the ground. In this way, he can sense the sound of approaching feet from a considerable distance. While he rests, his senses maintain contact with the immediate environment. This contact keeps him aware of potential danger and allows him to sleep peacefully.

He returned to the earlier question. What happens to you when you get nightmares? Your mind travels to a faraway place . . . a land of pure fear, a world made of thoughts totally disconnected from where you are, the here and now. Connecting to your senses is a way to emerge from this illusion. In doing so, you can more effectively evaluate any real threats. Your mind and body will react accordingly, and when things are safe you will rest. This can help you to have nice dreams.

## Managing Frightening Visions

This San healer's approach to fear and nightmares was strangely similar to what I later learned with the Shipibos. In ayahuasca ceremony, participants sometimes encounter nightmarish visions and feel as though they have been transported to a land of pure fear. This can be overwhelming and sometimes they need help. Shipibo shamans help such individuals through song, by singing icaros to them. In addition to their vibrational and energetic qualities, the icaros have words. In the Shipibo tradition, the lyrics of the icaros are largely improvised to address in real time what is going on with the participant.

Years later, Ricardo taught me to sing to people's five senses to help them through frightening visions. In the icaros, the shaman sings to strengthen and center the participant's five senses. This helps to calm the mind. The shaman can then sing to further center the mind and reconnect it to the channel that leads to the heart and eventually to all of the energy centers. The goal is to reconnect the individual's mind to the five senses and the internal sense: how you feel inside your body, your heart, your gut, and throughout. This sense is called interoception. These internal sensations inform us about the physiologic condition of our body. We also experience our emotions through these sensations.

In fear or in negative thinking, we can become trapped in our minds. As the San healer described, left to its own devices the mind can carry us to a "faraway place," disconnected from our surroundings and from our bodies. This can make it very difficult to feel safe and relaxed. An overactive mind that is disconnected from the senses and the body can get lost in narrow-minded, repetitive thought. Out-of-control repetitive thinking underlies certain mental health problems like depression, anxiety, addiction, and Obsessive Compulsive Disorder (OCD). In anxiety, fearful thoughts dominate. In depression, for example, negative and hopeless thoughts dominate.

## The Default Mode Network

Antidepressants helped me find relief from repetitive negative thinking and allowed me to reconnect to the outside world, to appreciate a nice day. Peyote quieted my mind in a much more profound and impactful way. There are some new theories about how antidepressants and psychedelic medicines might do this. Both forms of medicine affect the serotonin system in a way that helps to modulate the function of a brain network known as the Default Mode Network (DMN).[1-7]

Overactivity of certain regions of this network is correlated to decreased awareness of the outside world and the body (interoception/emotional awareness). Such DMN overactivity is associated with narrow and repetitive thinking patterns. Just as open-minded thinking is associated with optimism, close-minded thinking is associated with pessimism.[5]

Overactivity in the DMN has been correlated to a variety of mental health conditions, including depression, anxiety, addiction, and Obsessive-Compulsive Disorder (OCD).[3,5] Each of these conditions is related to narrow and repetitive thinking patterns and a disconnection from the outside world and from one's feelings. Antidepressants are, with varying results, used to treat each of these four conditions, likely because of their effects on DMN activity.[2,3] Psychedelic medicines such as LSD, psilocybin, and ayahuasca have also shown promise in the treatment of depression, anxiety, addiction, and OCD.[5-11]

Transcending limited thinking patterns is essential in overcoming depression and the above-mentioned disorders. Emotional trauma and excessive stress (from, for example, medical school) scar the mind, reducing access to creativity, feeling, and the world around us. During dreamlike psychedelic experiences, like my Spirit Walk, gates in the mind are re-opened, allowing for "open-hearted free-flowing emotional experiences and heightened sensory awareness."[5] Psychedelic medicines and in fact spiritual practice, e.g., meditation, can help expand thinking beyond maladaptive patterns.[2-14] This expansion in consciousness is essential in spiritual and emotional healing, as it allows the mind to re-open to the heart.

That night around the fire, our friend the San healer reminded us to stay connected to our senses for peace of mind. Back in the Kalahari, he and his colleagues had faced grave danger on multiple occasions, but they didn't look anxious, depressed, or preoccupied. As one connects to the present, outwardly and within, the mind calms. Peyote guided me out of depression by helping me to reconnect. In order to stay healthy, though, I would need to find ways to maintain this connection.

Open-minded spiritual practices like meditation are a more stable pathway to expanded consciousness. As there are continued stresses, the mind will need continued maintenance. Meditation is a slower pathway, but its effects are longer lasting than psychedelics. In my experience, service as a spiritual practice can also bolster mental health. Without some form of integration, emotional support, and/or new behavior, even the most enlightening psychedelic experience will wane into a mere temporary shift in thinking. However, in the short term, such an experience may give someone the boost they need to find a more stable path.

Strangely enough, as I discovered myself, this psychedelic boost (involving alterations in DMN activity and expanded consciousness) can quite often induce a mystical experience. Mystical experiences can profoundly alter our sense of meaning and purpose, which brings us back to the subject of ayahuasca.[15-16]

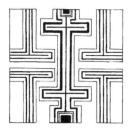

# CHAPTER 6

# Tukuymanta

In the mid-1800s, Richard Spruce and Alexander von Humboldt were two of the first European explorers to encounter the aya-huasca decoction. These early explorers reported hearing tales of the beverage's magical effects: stories of visions, "out-of-body travel," predictions of the future, location of lost objects, and contact with the dead. Upon experimentation, these explorers verified the tea's mystical properties.

— Rick Strassman MD, *DMT: The Spirit Molecule*

In 2006, I completed Family Medicine Residency and, as described in Chapter 2, in 2007 I took my first trip to Peru with Keyvan. I had my first ayahuasca experience, and then I had two more very profound ceremonies on that visit as well. Each time the experience was more familiar. After the third ceremony it was time to go. I wept that day. I wept in gratitude. I felt like those ceremonies had brought me "back" to a connection with the South American soil. Even though I was born in the United States, my spirit had always felt somehow displaced. The Shipibos had somehow reconnected me to my roots and to the Earth. I did not realize how much I was aching for that connection. A calling began to stir within me.

After Peru, the fellowship then travelled merrily, merrily down the river to Brazil. It was an incredible journey down the Amazon. There was fun to be had and plenty of time to contemplate my experiences in Peru. Once the adventure was complete, I headed back to Los Angeles, knowing that one day I would return to the rainforest. First though, I would need to develop my medical career.

During residency I had been moonlighting in the urgent care clinic at a large HMO (Health Maintenance Organization). I continued to work there after residency and started some shifts in its primary care clinic. I worked part-time so that I could continue to explore my interests in integrative medicine.

I was also curious about research. I had continued exploring the integration of Traditional Chinese Medicine and allopathic medicine at UCLA and had also been doing independent research into a form of light therapy. Dr. Sandra Daley, a Panamanian-American powerhouse, one of my mentors and another angel from my medical training, had been encouraging me to pursue academic work. She helped me to find funding for an opportunity back at the UCSD School of Medicine, and so, after the initial Fellowship of the River, in mid-2007 I moved back down to San Diego to enter a bona fide postdoctoral research fellowship in the department of psychiatry. This research fellowship introduced me to the academic study of mind-body medicine. Mind-body medicine examines the way in which thoughts and emotions influence physical health. I spent two years in research at UCSD. This work informed and guided my subsequent studies in what Ricardo's colleagues referred to as "Amazonian psychiatry."

At UCSD, I worked under Dr. Paul Mills in the division of Behavioral Medicine. He is a long-standing National Institute of Health (NIH)-supported clinical investigator with expertise in psychoneuroimmune processes in wellness and in disease. Psychoneuroimmunology (PNI), also referred to as psychoneuroendocrine immunology (PNEI), is the study of the interaction between psychological processes and the nervous, immune, and endocrine systems of the body. In 2007, Paul's lab was running a number of studies investigating such things as how exercise affects inflammation in the cardiovascular system and how depression affects cardiovascular disease. PNI and PNEI are essentially the study of the mechanisms underlying the so-called mind-body connection.

Paul is a spiritual man and an advanced meditator. His initial doctoral research was on the effects of meditation on the autonomic nervous system and the immune system at the Maharishi University in Iowa. Paul has been one of my major academic influences and spiritual teachers. During my research fellowship, he was in his mid-fifties, a tall slender man with deep blue eyes. One look into his gaze and you can see that he likes to paddle out into the deep end of human consciousness.

While working for Paul at the lab, I had the opportunity to attend a few academic conferences. In 2008, I went to the Scripps Center for Integrative Medicine conference on natural supplements. I remember going to a talk on the herbal medicines of the world. The lecture reviewed available research on traditional plant medicines. This one-hour PowerPoint presentation managed to cover a lot of territory.

When it came to the topics of Traditional Chinese Medicine and Ayurvedic Medicine from India, the slides just kept coming and coming, herb after herb. But when it came time to discuss Traditional Amazonian Plant Medicine, there was only one slide to share. On the screen was a photo of a donkey pulling a cart so full of cluttered plants that their weight had actually see-sawed the donkey into the air, feet dangling. There was no further information given, just too many plants for one donkey. On closer inspection, I could see that the photo was not even taken in South America; the people standing around the cart, by their dress, appeared to be South Asians. As a Colombian-American doctor interested in natural medicines, I was embarrassed.

True, there has been a paucity of placebo-controlled double-blind studies in the jungle, but just one slide with a donkey? I knew that Amazonian plant medicine warranted more discussion. I had seen some of what those plant medicines could do. My grandfather's best friend had built his career studying traditional Amazonian plant medicines.

My maternal grandfather's name was José "Pepe" M. Palomares-Bernal. His best friend, a man named Hernando Garcia-Barriga, was a medical botanist based in Bogotá, Colombia. Dr. Garcia had made a name for himself in the 1940s by traveling on horseback to the Colombian Amazon to study with native tribes. His extended time with indigenous healers led to a very productive academic career. He became a preeminent scholar in botany and plant medicines. Dr. Garcia helped to found the first botanical institute in Colombia and the first botanical garden. Later in his career in 1974, he published the three volume text *Flora Medicinal de Colombia*, a definitive work in its time. As my mother had often reminded me, Dr. Garcia had even received special recognition from Harvard.

My *abuelito* (grandfather) Pepe passed away when I was very young, when we were in the United States. Every couple of years we would visit Bogotá and Medellín in Colombia to spend time with our grandparents, aunts, uncles, and cousins. In Bogotá, my mother always tried to make sure we visited Hernando Garcia and his family, so that they might teach us something about our grandfather, his lifelong friend.

In addition to his work at the university, Dr. Garcia had also developed his own brand of herbal medicines. Those plant medicines had helped my younger brother through childhood asthma and had also helped other friends and family members through a variety of ailments. As I grew older and my mother saw that I was interested in "alternative" medicines, she tried to encourage me to pay more attention to Dr. Garcia and his work. At the time, I had not imagined that I would one day become so interested in Amazonian shamanism.

Growing up primarily in Phoenix, I did not think about Hernando Garcia very often. Over the years, we visited him a few times and I remember him as an older man, friendly and gracious. At his family's apartment, I remember seeing ocelot skins on the walls and samples of exotic plants scattered around.

Somewhere along the way, on television or something, I had heard of *yagé*, the Colombian version of ayahuasca. On one of those visits, as a teenager, I asked Hernando Garcia about the *yagé*. He really wouldn't say much about it to me. He just mumbled something discouraging about the poor nutrition of the tribes, that I shouldn't romanticize their lifestyle. That was all I got from him. Dr. Garcia passed away in 2005 at the age of 92. Back home in Arizona, from time to time I would see his books on the shelf in my dad's office.

During that presentation at the conference, I was reminded of Dr. Garcia. I mentioned this to Dr. Paul Mills. Paul was curious about my experiences in the Amazon and was generally supportive of my interest in ayahuasca shamanism. I set aside some vacation time from the lab to head back down to Iquitos on my own, this time for two weeks. I wanted to go deeper into the world of the plants.

Nearly a year after my first visit, I flew back to Iquitos. It was good to be back and to step out of the plane into the warm jungle air. Another mototaxi driver was waiting for me. He drove me directly out to the same healing center. I was hoping to see Ricardo again, but this time, the maestro was working with a different assistant shaman, one of his more experienced apprentices, Rolando Tangoa Murayari. Rolando is a little rougher around the edges than Ricardo and is for some reason missing all of his upper incisors. He loves telling jokes, and his distinctive smile is joyfully punctuated by his canines. Laughter, he says, is the most spiritually interesting subject. He is an intelligent man and a dedicated healer whomI have gotten to know more and more over the years.

Rolando grew up in the rustic outskirts of Pucallpa with his many, many siblings, some of whom have gone on to professional careers in politics and engineering. Like many Amazonian natives, he is from an area that floods during the Amazonian winter (the wet season). His parents' house is planted on stilts, and in the rainy season, their humble home doubles as a dock for small canoes. He swears that his mom, a Cocama native, has trained their jungle dog, during the high water, to carefully go to the bathroom over the edge of one of the canoes. Anything less would be uncivilized. At that time, he was in his early 40s, a couple of years younger than Ricardo. Rolando was in fact the key person that set Ricardo on his shamanic path, having led him through a month-long treatment years ago.

I had a brought a hammock as a gift for Ricardo, but as he was not there I gave it to Rolando. We quickly became friends. Rolando was often communicating with the *pasajeros*, and he asked me to help with translation. You'll recall that I had also translated a bit for Ricardo and the other shamans. I was eager to help out, as this was always an opportunity for me to get to know the shamans more intimately. At that time, this center was running six ceremonies per week, and guests had two options for their stay. For one price you could participate in ayahuasca ceremonies every other night, or for an added price you could participate in all six ceremonies per week. This was an unusually intense schedule and a unique opportunity.

I signed up for the twelve ceremonies, Sunday through Friday for two weeks. Again I took the *vomitivo* and started my traditional Shipibo *dieta*. I met with the shamans to explain my intentions. I was prescribed a mix of plants to help me regain vitality after my prolonged medical training. This mix was known as "*21 plantas*." Instead of staying in one of the guest rooms, I decided to try one of the jungle tambos (huts). To go deeper with the plants, isolation is encouraged during the diet, so that you don't mix your energies with others. As the peyote church had taught me, social contact stimulates your ego and personality, sometimes at the expense of deeper spiritual exploration. The tambo would offer me greater seclusion.

This jungle tambo was an open-air structure in the forest situated along one of the many trails on their extensive property. It was composed of a thatched roof over a patch of dirt and included a bed with a mosquito net, a hammock, and a small wooden table. It was a brief walk from the rest of the center, not far from the bathrooms, showers, kitchen, dining area, and lounge, but it did offer me a place to go to be alone.

The center was full of guests and sometimes they split the ceremony into two ceremonies, one at the main maloka and another at a large wooden house. Night after night, these ceremonies were a rip-roaring icaro-filled extravaganza. Strange and mysterious experiences were the norm. In the day, I spent my free time socializing with the other *pasajeros*, sharing experiences and talking to the shamans.

Otherwise I would hang out at my tambo, resting and reflecting. Out in the forest, the bugs were generally worse and so I spent most of my time on the bed, resting within the safety of the mosquito net.

Day after day, as soon as night came, it was once again time for another ceremony. Every night is different with ayahuasca, every ceremony unique. Over the first week, I sat in six ceremonies. Every night I seemed to go a little further, expanding my exploration of the world of ayahuasca. I was learning a lot during the day—through translating for the shamans, from their guidance, and from the varied experiences of the other *pasajeros*. As I moved into the second week, my ceremonies became increasingly visual.

# Between Two Worlds

At the ninth ceremony (my twelfth ayahuasca experience), I had my first experience between two worlds. I was sitting up on my mat listening. The shamans were singing on the other side of the maloka. The ceremonial space was pitch black. My vision opened. Initially I saw a white, intricately embroidered veil flowing in front of me. Behind it children were playing. This was the invitation. Dancing shadows behind the veil. The veil opened and suddenly I realized that I was sitting in some kind of brightly lit living room. This living room was overlaid onto my reality in the dark maloka. It was my first three-dimensional ayahuasca vision and it surrounded me, like some kind of parallel universe, Star Trek holodeck-style.

As I turned my head to survey the maloka, I would also pan the visual space of this other dimension. I could look up, down, and all around. I was seated in a fancy living room; it felt like my grandmother's apartment in Bogotá, formally arranged, except this was a cosmic grandmother or perhaps it was the grandmother ayahuasca, or some combination of all of the above. In the visions, I was seated on a comfortable white couch. It felt as if there were other spirits there waiting, but I could not sense them for sure. It was as if we were waiting for an audience with this grandmother. She was somewhere down a hallway at the other end of the room beyond another veil.

From time to time, everything would shimmer with a pulse of energy that would send subtle designs rippling over the surfaces of everything in the room. All of the walls and furniture were bright white. On one wall to the left was a large piece of artwork, portraying a golden crocodile surfacing from a red background. In solid gold bas-relief, the head, back, and tail floated over a flat, red, velvety surface, curving in mid-swim. On another wall was a multicolored crystal light fixture, a sort of posing snake bust, glowing pink, blue, and violet. There were other couches for sitting and a large white coffee table. I waited and enjoyed the inviting atmosphere. It seemed as if someone were going to be serving refreshments, tea or something. It was welcoming, but I never did meet anyone directly. I looked around. Intricate light designs again pulsed over the scenery. Eventually the room faded into darkness. I laid back to listen and contemplate.

As Rolando had explained, my diet was helping to clean me and further opened me to the visionary realms. The recurrent ceremonies, the plants, and the icaros opened me more and more to the spiritual dimension. By the tenth ceremony of the series, I had been dieting for 10 days or so. The night before, I had experienced a 3-D virtual reality but I had been unable to leave my body to enter further. I was fixed to my mat and could not see beyond that veil at the other end of the room. On the tenth ceremony night, Wednesday, ayahuasca invited me back into the visionary world.

It started like all of the other nights. Sit quietly and respectfully. Go up and receive the ayahuasca. Meditate on your intentions for the ceremony. Smoke a mapacho in the dark and wait for things to open up. After some time, the ceremony got underway. Multiple shamans were singing, but Rolando's song seemed to be leading. His icaro captured my focus. Rolando's chants come from deep within his being and sometimes have a sorrowful quality. This particular song was more vibrant.

As I had been advised, I was concentrating on the icaro, his icaro, tuning in to his medicine, allowing it to enter and influence my world. A new vision opened up; a dirt path appeared in front of me.

Without thinking, deep in the *mareación*, my spirit sprung up out of my body and began to walk down this path. On both sides of the path, illuminated from below, were many colorful plants of all shapes and sizes. I did not distinguish any particular plant. For me it was a path through diverse jungle scenery. As in the night scenes of the film *Avatar*, the plants seemed awake, glowing pink and purple.

As I wandered down this meandering path, I approached Rolando, closing in on his voice on the other side of the maloka. At one point I was standing in front of him and I could see him clearly. He was sitting up with his head bent down, concentrated in his chant. His body had transformed into that of a big cat, like a lion or jaguar, with smooth, red-colored fur. He was resting on his haunches. His head had become that of a large black anaconda, eyes peering, deeply focused as he crooned on, singing his icaro. Surrounding this dark snakehead was a large mane of huge yellow flower petals. His song drew me in. Rhythmic and mystical, it was penetrating my mind.

I stood back in awe as this snake-flower-lion-shaman sang his icaro. Just as I got comfortable, one of the extra-large flower petals leapt from his head and pushed forward into my face. The song continued, and the flower petal quickly dominated my visual field. The yellow petal then morphed into a large green leaf. With digital precision, bright lights traced its every vein into existence. With increasing intensity, the leaf's shape, its gestalt, its cells, its molecules, all of its defining characteristics were burned into my mind.

In a culminating flash, a voice spoke softly, "Joe . . . you have not been paying attention. These plants that I have shown you are real plants. If you would only ask, you might learn something . . . Tomorrow you will find this leaf."

The vision dissipated and I realized I was back on my mat. Rolando and the other shamans were still singing on the other side.

I had heard that the shamans learn about medicinal plants in ayahuasca visions. I was very excited as it seemed something like that was happening to me.

Once the ceremony ended, I left the maloka and headed to bed. I walked the fifty yards or so down the trail to my tambo, guided by my flashlight. I crawled into bed under the mosquito net, flipped off the flashlight, and lay back. I closed my eyes and smiled. It was time to rest. In the pitch darkness, I fell asleep amidst the jungle symphony.

The next morning, I woke up with the intuition and the hope that I would find the leaf from my vision. I stepped into my flip-flops and headed down the trail back toward the dining hall for breakfast. It was still cool out and the morning light was coming down through the trees. I glanced at the plants along the way, looking for signs of anything familiar. After only a few paces I found it. There it was, a small weed along the trail. I had seen this plant many times before. It has very distinct red flowers resembling the Rolling Stones-style "hot lips." I doubted myself. It was probably just my hope, my imagination. My intuition however was very sure. The leaves were the same, exactly like the one I had seen the night before. The red flower petals were bold and almost plastic, with a yellow center, like the colors from my vision. I picked a leaf and took it with me to breakfast.

On my way there, I ran into the master shaman. I told him what had happened and showed him the green leaf. From ten feet away he identified it as *beso de la novia,* meaning "kiss of the girlfriend" in Spanish, named for its hot-lips flowers. I asked him what they used it for, and he explained that the Shipibos sometimes mixed this plant into their *curare* mixture (beso de la novia is *Psychotria poeppigiana,* a close cousin of the chacruna). Made in a variety of forms by Amazonian tribes, curare is a plant-based poison used traditionally for hunting game.

My ears perked up. This was odd. In medical school, the Amazonian shamans were really only mentioned in one context: the discovery of muscle paralytics. Western scientists and doctors learned about muscle paralytics, the kind that are used in surgery, from the Amazonian shamans. The curare dart poison contains alkaloids that paralyze skeletal muscles by interfering with nerve transmission to those muscles. In the Amazon, curare poisons are made from source plants and are used to hunt game high in the trees, like monkeys.

For example, with a blowgun, a native hunter fires a poisoned dart at a monkey. The dart poison blocks nerve transmission to the monkey's skeletal muscles, including those of the arms and legs. The monkey's muscles go limp and it falls to the ground. The poison can also paralyze the diaphragm muscle, stopping breathing. The curare poison does not necessarily kill the monkeys. It leaves them limp and they fall from the trees. Although the fall is dangerous, the monkey might survive. Either way, once poisoned, that monkey will be finished off by the hunter, cooked, and eaten (curare can be safely ingested orally as it is not absorbed by the gastrointestinal tract).

When Western scientists got samples of this poisonous plant mixture, they began to experiment. I heard one story in which they poisoned a donkey (different donkey, by the way) with curare and then learned that they could keep this poisoned donkey alive by using a bellows to ventilate its paralyzed lungs. After some time, the poison wore off and the donkey's muscles returned to normal function. The donkey stood up and walked away. This temporary paralysis proved to be quite useful in the operating room and hospital. From the curare, several muscle paralytics have since been derived.

These muscle paralytics contributed to a revolution in surgical possibilities. Prior anesthesia regimens sometimes required life-threatening doses to keep the patient from reacting reflexively to the scalpels. But with curare-derived paralytics, as long as respiratory support is maintained, you do not have to put people under so deeply before cutting them open. Anesthesia is administered independently from the paralytic/relaxant, and both can be adjusted independently to reduce toxicity. Among other things, this breakthrough gave rise to horror movies about anesthesia awareness in which paralyzed patients are operated on while wide awake. But most importantly, Amazonian curare led to overall improvements in the safety of surgical anesthesia and allowed for a quantum leap in surgical practice.

As a medical doctor I was taken aback when I heard this Amazonian shaman mention curare in response to my questions. The leaf vision was impressive on its own, but curare? This was not a simple coincidence. Surprised, I was left thinking. The shaman went on about his way.

# Family Connection

After a few more ceremonies, I headed back to California and immediately began telling my friends and family about my experiences in Iquitos. I kept thinking, someone needs to make a documentary about this mystical medicine.

On a visit to LA, I talked to my friend Fred, a documentary producer for the Discovery Channel. He was interested in my experience and also curious about the phenomenon of ayahuasca tourism. But he was busy with other projects and made it clear that we would really have to do our homework before considering taking such a project further. We would need to review existing ayahuasca documentaries and see if they had not already covered similar territory.

Fred did some research and gave me names of a few films to review. In particular, he was interested in one called *Peyote to LSD: The Psychedelic Odyssey*. At the time, it was available only on the History channel, and I didn't have cable in my apartment in San Diego. Then oddly enough, one day a few weeks later while visiting my parents in Arizona, we were flipping channels on the television and there it was. Not only was this a pleasant surprise, it was a chance to share some of what I had been investigating with my parents. As you might imagine, they were not exactly thrilled to learn that their son, whom they had put through medical school, was drifting back south to the Amazon to drink hallucinogenic tea with indigenous shamans. The documentary gave them an opportunity to learn about visionary plant medicine in a respectful and academic context.

*Peyote to LSD: The Psychedelic Odyssey* is a documentary about the life of Harvard ethnobotanist Richard Evans Schultes. It is narrated/presented by his former student Wade Davis, author of, among other things, *One River*, which is in part a biography of Schultes' life. Schultes lived from 1915 to 2001 and was an ethnobotanical pioneer and an inspirational professor. In *One River*, Davis describes a period during which Dr. Schultes kept a basket of peyote buttons sitting in front of his office door as an optional laboratory assignment. This was of course well before peyote was considered a controlled substance.

Before watching this film, I had never heard of Richard Evans Schultes, and I sat there on my parents' couch, mesmerized. As I would learn from the film that day, Dr. Schultes had had a unique academic career as an ethnobotanist. His undergraduate thesis was on the ceremonial use of peyote among the Kiowa natives in Oklahoma. His field research included participating in multiple Kiowa peyote ceremonies. His doctoral thesis explored traditional psychedelic plant and fungi use in Oaxaca, Mexico and involved similar fieldwork. I was surprised to learn about all of his accomplishments and his profound interest in plant shamanism.

He was among the first scientists to explore psychedelics and collaborated extensively with the aforementioned Swiss chemist Albert Hoffman (who discovered LSD). In 1942, Schultes was sent to conduct research in the Colombian Amazon. It was World War II and the Allies were looking for new sources of rubber for tires and for other natural Amazonian resources. Schultes travelled to the Amazon to investigate South American rubber and concurrently secured funding to pursue his own ethnobotanical research. This work gave him a chance to follow in the footsteps of his hero, 1800s Amazonian explorer Richard Spruce, who had reported on the ayahuasca decoction. Schultes would continue his personal exploration into ceremonial psychoactive plant use. In the Colombian Amazon, he participated in many master plant ceremonies.

Among his tasks, as part of a fellowship with the National Research Council, Schultes was charged with identifying the source plants of the curare poison. Although Western scientists had accessed curare preparations, they still needed to identify the source plants in order to isolate key alkaloids. With his experience with indigenous Native American cultures, Schultes was the ideal man for the job. His enthusiasm for shamanic plant medicine also seems to have helped him get in with the locals.

Schultes is credited with many ethnobotanical discoveries. However, I was most interested to learn that Schultes is the American credited with identifying the curare source plants, allowing for the subsequent expansion in surgical practice. He was also the first scientist to academically examine ayahuasca. There I was watching cable at my parents' house. Curare . . . again, and I remembered the leaf in my visions and the words of the shaman.

I made my way back to San Diego and to the lab. I looked up my good friend Chris, a devout spiritualist and academic researcher and self-proclaimed paradigm angel. He likes to anonymously connect like-minded researchers in order to help them expand their paradigms. Chris has a little over twenty years on me and he experienced the sixties. He had also taught me about the first wave of psychedelic academic research and was very curious about my adventures in the Amazon. I mentioned the leaf vision and how I had stumbled upon Schultes. He was shocked to learn that I was only just then becoming aware of Schultes and his work.

"You've got to get his books. Study them. Take them to the Amazon and study them with the shamans!" he advised.

I ordered some used copies on Amazon, including *The Plants of the Gods,* which is co-written by Schultes and Hoffman, *One River* by Wade Davis, and some of Schultes's more academic works. As I looked through Schultes's work, I noticed that he frequently referred to Colombian botanist Dr. Hernando Garcia! This was surprising, but it did make sense. My abuelito's friend and Schultes, the two university botanists in Colombia, were contemporaries.

Then one night I was in my apartment alone, working on an art piece for my brother Mario. This piece was inspired by my maternal grandfather Pepe's grandmother Rafaela Bernal. They say she was a mystical woman. I was quietly arranging some images for a collage on the brown shag carpet in my bedroom. The Schultes books were strewn across the floor nearby. It was quiet, no music, just quiet.

Then, suddenly, for the first time in my life, I felt the presence of my grandfather Pepe. My abuelito Pepe spoke to me. It was an invisible presence, a breeze of a thought that blew into my mind and said, "Joe, Schultes was friends with Hernando Garcia; he was our friend."

Just as the yellow flower petal had transformed into the leaf, rapidly crystallized from all of its atomic parts, this story materialized.

My grandfather was Hernando Garcia's best friend. Schultes was Hernando Garcia's close colleague. They were all good friends.

I saw my copy of *One River* on the floor. I just knew that Garcia would be in the index. I opened the book, and, sure enough, there he was on page 204, "his colleague and friend" and "the only other botanist to have worked in Sibundoy (the homeland of a well-established indigenous community)."[1]

In all our visits, Hernando Garcia never had much to say about ayahuasca to me. Schultes himself, after countless ceremonies, publicly reported that he had only seen colors. Later, after all of this was revealed, I started reading more about Hernando Garcia and his illustrious career. On the topic of ayahuasca shamans, in 1958 Garcia wrote that "savage Indians who have never left their forests and who, of course, can have no idea of civilized life, describe, in their particular language, and with more or less precision, the details of houses, castles, and cities peopled by multitudes."[2]

Before drinking ayahuasca, before the diet and the plants and the icaros, I had never heard of Richard Evans Schultes. The plants directed my attention to him, in this very mysterious way. This is one example of how the plants teach. What was the award that Hernando Garcia had received from Harvard, the one my mom had always tried to tell me about? I looked it up; it was the Richard Evans Schultes Award. Hernando Garcia's son Darrio verified to me that Dr. Schultes was an intimate friend of the Garcia family. In later discussions, Darrio explained that many of the famous photos taken of Schultes deep in the Colombian Amazon were in fact taken by his father Hernando. I can imagine them all having a coffee somewhere in Bogotá: Richard, Hernando, and Pepe.

Hernando Garcia is the unsung Colombian hero in the curare story, overlooked, just like the indigenous masters who taught him, and who taught Schultes. Western culture and modern Latin-American culture have largely disregarded the knowledge and wisdom of indigenous traditions. Few academics have humbled themselves in order to learn the traditional way alongside Amazonian shamans. Schultes and Garcia respectfully studied with

Amazonian masters. Both went on to stellar careers in botany and ethnobotany.

After this mysterious revelation, I realized that I also wanted to be a bridge between two worlds, Western science and indigenous shamanism. I wanted to embrace my cultural heritage and study in a traditional setting under Amazonian shamans. I decided to follow the example of my grandfather's best friend. This decision put my medical school difficulties into a new context. The basic science education that I'd always resisted in fact gave me a unique perspective into how to combine those worlds. I continued work at the lab and I continued returning to the Amazon.

In 2009, I had the honor of presenting this curare story to a small gathering organized by my aunt in Bogotá, the Tukuymanta Conference (*tukuymanta,* I was told, means something like "well-being" in the Quechua language). Paul Mills, Hernando's son Darrio Garcia, and a master Shipibo shaman all participated. It was a wonderful conference that inspired a lot of interesting discussion. It was also a chance for me to express my respect for the ancestral medicine of our land. There is still not enough dialogue between academic scholars and traditional men and women of knowledge. Unfortunately, remnants of Spanish colonialism still linger in the Latin-American consciousness, including a shame and prejudice over indigenous roots. It is my belief that Latin America should take pride in its powerful indigenous knowledge, which of course includes the practice of Traditional Amazonian Plant Medicine.

# CHAPTER 7

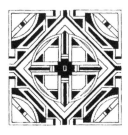

# Responsible Practice

*Be careful what you wish for.*

—anonymous

Traditional Amazonian Plant Medicine is built upon cultural experience and wisdom. This wisdom is rooted in a reverence and respect for the master plants, teaching plants that have been used and identified over many generations. Most of these plants have only subtle effects on the mind. Ayahuasca tea, however, is highly psychoactive and must be approached very carefully, as there are risks involved. Ayahuasca tourists who come seeking powerful visionary experiences sometimes prioritize these experiences over their own healing. Many get more than what they bargained for, and some are pushed over the edge.

Although a competent shaman should be able to guide participants through even the most mind-blowing experiences, one should not ignore the possibility of unforeseen circumstances. Wisdom reminds us to be careful and to learn from the experience of others.

During that two-week stay at the center where I had the vision of the curare plant, I got to know a few of my fellow *pasajeros*. There was a younger Frenchman named Jean, thin and intelligent with a big

59

head of sandy dreadlocks. When it came to ayahuasca, he was hungry for more, more, more—wanting to push the experience further.

At the ceremonies, the shamans served the ayahuasca at their own discretion but were generally open to increasing one's dose if appropriate. Jean kept making the case for drinking more, but Rolando disagreed. But as Jean continued to ask for more, night after night, Rolando finally decided to let him find what he was looking for. However, Rolando made it clear that the consequences would be Jean's own responsibility, not the shamans.

As I have since heard the shamans say in similar situations, as Rolando served Jean he said, "*castigate,*" punish yourself. (Rolando had, in truth, already determined that Jean could safely handle the higher dose. If necessary, Rolando would help Jean, but on principle, he would first let him suffer and learn.)

Once again we waited for the effect to kick in. That night, Jean was sitting on the mat to my right. Things got going. I myself had a very powerful experience and for an extended period was not able to move or speak. I could however turn my head a bit and noticed that Jean was writhing, appearing pained. He moaned quietly and then later managed to crawl to the front of his mat. There, hunched over on the wood, he was assuming all kinds of strange postures. He was for the most part quiet, staring far, far way into an apparently terrifying space.

As usual, the ceremony went on for hours. Things had smoothed out for me, but I was not sure about Jean. As soon as it was over, Jean, looking rather shaken, quietly exited. After some chitchat with Rolando and the others, I wandered out to check on the young Frenchman.

Jean had gone back to his single room. In the distance I could see him sitting there with a candle. As I approached in the dark with my flashlight, he called out, "Joe!" I was still twenty yards away, but he knew it was me. His senses were wide open and his intuition was in overdrive. He had just been through one of the most terrifying experiences of his life.

He invited me into the room. "I knew it was you," he said. "I was trying to call out to you for help during the ceremony," he continued.

I explained that I had sensed he was in trouble, but that at the time I was incapable of offering help. I had been unable to make even a sound, much less talk to him.

He described how the ayahuasca had hit him like a freight train. As planned, Rolando and the shamans had left him to his experience. Before he knew it, Jean had transformed into a lizard and was lost in what he described as a very base consciousness. He had lost complete control. He was reduced to lizard being and lizard behavior. His ego and identity had been completely shattered. This went on for an apparent eternity. Terrified and lost, he was at the mercy of *la Madre* Ayahuasca and her cruel tutelage.

After enduring the lizard experience, Jean was then transformed into a number of forms and ultimately reduced to a helpless puddle of energy pooled on the maloka floor. He spent the rest of the night trying to grasp what had happened. For some time afterward, he did notice that the experience had somehow opened a kind of extrasensory perception.

The next day he slowly recovered, and over time he began to integrate the experience. People have many different kinds of experiences with ayahuasca. Shamanically speaking, once must be very careful as energetic realms are revealed under the influence of the medicine. In the ceremony, some receive information or see extraordinary things. For others the experience is purely physical, without visions. On other occasions the experience can be very dark and upsetting, even terrifying.

When I was translating for Rolando with the *pasajeros*, we would discuss difficult ayahuasca experiences like Jean's and other more personal journeys. A recurrent line of questioning and complaining came from the guests.

"Why is this coming up in my ayahuasca ceremony?"

"I don't want to see this."

"I thought I was over that."

"I thought I had put that behind me. Where are the beautiful visions?"

I have often repeated Rolando's response to similar questions. Rolando did not learn about ayahuasca during a brief vacation in the Amazon. As an Amazonian *ayahuasquero,* he learned from the experience of multiple generations within his own family and community. He was a bit surprised to hear these kinds of questions over and over. He noted that gringos always wanted nice visions. Perhaps they did not understand, perhaps the ayahuasca is not for them. Dark visions are part of the experience, even for advanced practitioners, even for those who say they are completely over all of their issues. The advanced practitioner must learn to navigate through these experiences and the related fear and doubt.

Rolando then described to me what it was like to become widely known as a shaman and to start working with foreigners. People he did not know started to evaluate him, to talk about him, to leave comments on the Internet about him. People started watching him more and more closely. Because he was involved in spiritual healing, they expected him to be perfect. And when he fell short, as anyone would, they criticized him freely, sometimes saying very cruel things.

This for him was like enduring dark ayahuasca visions. He had to learn to weather the blows of negativity. Eventually, he discovered that no matter what people said, he did not need to suffer. Instead, he needed to learn to say thank you.

Why thank you? Because what those people were saying was probably true. And if it was true, then it was true a few minutes earlier, before he had ever heard it, when he was feeling fine, when he was smiling. Nothing had actually changed. It's the same truth as before. He says thank you because their criticism and negativity have helped him to become more aware.

The darkness opens our awareness, Rolando observes, and for this we should be grateful. Jean learned this the hard way.

## Shamanic Plant Medicine Is Not for Everyone

Jean made it through his very frightening experience and, ultimately, gained an opportunity to raise his awareness and learn. Although sometimes overwhelming and seemingly "eternal," the *mareación* of ayahuasca usually settles down after a period of four or five hours.

This, however, is not always the case. Some intense ayahuasca experiences are neither safe nor productive.

During his rather shocking ayahuasca journey, Jean's ego completely dissolved. Researchers have correlated the experience of ego dissolution to psychedelically induced changes in the brain (namely in the DMN).[1] Such rapid ego dissolution can be very intense, and sometimes problematic. The ego serves to ground us, to help us to test reality, to plan and prevent uncertainty. If we are not well-prepared, rapid ego dissolution results in magical thinking, paranoia, and delusions. Open-minded thinking is healthy, but ungrounded thinking can be dangerous.

In people with a prior history of bipolar disorder, schizophrenia, and/or psychotic symptoms, the use of shamanic plant medicine is not currently recommended. Such individuals are particularly vulnerable to ayahuasca's mentally destabilizing effects, and ingesting it can cause prolonged and problematic alterations in consciousness.[2]

I am aware of a few cases in which ayahuasca pushed at-risk individuals into prolonged manic and psychotic states, lasting days and even weeks. Despite attempts to calm these individuals through traditional means, psychiatric medical intervention was ultimately necessary to bring them back down to baseline.

Although shamanic plant medicines are sacred, they are not for everyone. Both the patient and practitioner bear responsibility in the medical decision-making process. When weighing treatment options for any health problem, one must very carefully choose the appropriate modality, setting, and practitioner(s). That being said, utilized responsibly, ayahuasca and the master plants can be very therapeutic in a number of specific health conditions, including, for example, post-traumatic stress disorder (PTSD). In 2009, while leading my first group journey to the Amazon, I witnessed this firsthand.

CHAPTER 8

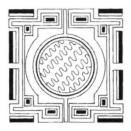

# Treating PTSD aboard Spaceship Earth

When people develop PTSD, the replaying of the trauma leads to sensitization: With every replay of the trauma there is an increasing level of distress. In those individuals, the traumatic event, which started out as a social and interpersonal process, develops secondary biological consequences that are hard to reverse once they become entrenched.

—Bessel van Der Kolk MD in *The Body Bears the Burden*

Start by doing what's necessary; then do what's possible; and suddenly you are doing the impossible.

—St. Francis of Assisi

After the Tukuymanta conference, I travelled back to Iquitos to meet up with a group of seekers I had organized for a ten-day program. We affectionately referred to this group as "Spaceship Earth," spinning off of a cosmic meme about Earth's journey through the galaxy. Spaceship Earth is also the name of a futuristic time machine experience at Disneyworld.

65

This was my fourth journey to Iquitos. There was the first trip with Keyvan in 2007, the second solo trip described in Chapters 6 and 7, and a third trip in 2008 with my friend CG, who wanted to see if the shamans could help him work through ongoing digestive problems and an emotionally traumatic upbringing. Ricardo Amaringo was there for that visit and was very helpful. We only had time for a seven-day experience; nonetheless, CG was very impressed. Before we left, the management at the center let me know that if I returned with a group of ten or more, my stay would be free. After returning to the United States, CG helped me to get the numbers I needed to "seed" Spaceship Earth.

Through a network of friends and friends of friends, a very interesting group assembled. There were ten participants in all, nine men and one woman, among them students, musicians, body workers, acupuncturists, educators, retirees, and even a young psychiatrist. The group included Miguel, who is my younger brother Camilo's father-in-law and a university professor from Phoenix and his close friend Russ, a retired healthcare administrator and combat veteran of the Vietnam War. Their presence was of particular significance to me, as Miguel is a close friend of my parents.

Spaceship Earth launched in the spring of 2009. I was in my second year of the research fellowship at UCSD and continued to work part-time as a family physician.

On my way over from Bogotá, I met up with a few "crew members" in Lima. The rest of the group came together in Iquitos, where our group program was to start on a Friday. Ricardo was back working at the center. Rolando had gone back to Pucallpa. As the main assistant shaman, Ricardo was also running ceremonies on his own and would handle some of our private group ceremonies.

Just as before, we prepared with the vomitive and started our *vegetalista* diets. In addition to the ayahuasca they would drink in ceremony, most of the group members were also assigned additional plants to assist them further in their healing process. I was planning to stay on past the group's departure to complete a one-month diet with the master plant coca (*Erythroxylum coca*).

A few of us had arrived at the center a few days early and had been invited to an additional ceremony on a Wednesday. This Wednesday ceremony turned out to be a dud. Despite drinking ayahuasca two and three times, no one felt much effect.

Although this dud ceremony served to quell first-time jitters among the newbies, it also left me concerned for my group's journey. I expressed my concerns to the treatment team and was told not to worry. I was assured that the ayahuasca would be "extra" strong for our Friday night ceremony. This I would come to learn meant that several crew members, four of the ten, would soil their pants. (This news was revealed the morning after, during the post-ceremonial discussion with the shamans. Ricardo laughed so hard, he actually fell out of his chair and rolled around on the ground. I had not seen anyone do that in a while.)

On Friday night, our private group gathered in the maloka, awaiting the arrival of the shamans. Although I was the most experienced participant on Spaceship Earth, my experiences had so far been few and far between. Excluding the dud ceremony, seven months had passed since my last trip to the jungle with CG.

The mood was light among the group. We were all settling into our spots, making a few jokes. Eventually, Ricardo opened the door and walked into the space. I was surprised to see him enter alone, as he usually worked with at least one assistant. He sat down on the mat next to me.

"Ricardo, what's the plan?" I said.

"Oh, we're going to drink ayahuasca and do the ceremony," he said.

"Yeah, but you're all alone. Who's going to help you?" I inquired.

"Oh, you're going to help me, Joe," he stated calmly. I did not like the sound of that.

"*I'm* going to help you? I have not been to a ceremony in seven months, I am not prepared, I don't think so, Ricardo," I said.

"Yes, Joe. You're going to help me," he restated.

I really wasn't sure what that meant. I felt a responsibility to the group but I did not know what he was expecting of me. I would have to wait and see. Ricardo served the ayahuasca and we all drank one by one. Ricardo drank last, again blowing his icaros into the glass before taking his dose. We all sat back and waited in the dark.

By that point I had drunk ayahuasca twenty or so times. I have since drunk many more times. Looking back though, that night was one of the strongest ayahuasca experiences I have ever had. I was, as we say, "super-*mareado*."

The ayahuasca came on very strong. When it is strong, it sometimes comes on all at once, with all of its force, *todo su fuerza*, in a tsunami of overwhelming energy. In this extremely altered state, one loses all sense of space and time. It can be very disorienting. We dissolve into a much larger universe and often lose the ability to describe our experience.

Once the ayahuasca effect came over me, I could not make out much of what was happening around me. I don't remember too much about the beginning. It was clear from all of the moaning that many in the group were sick and vomiting. Despite the messy scene, Ricardo somehow maintained his composure.

In the throes of my overwhelming experience, his shamanic presence appeared supernatural. He sat and observed, quietly, then began to sing. After a few early icaros, Ricardo called me over to sit in front of him. He was planning to sing to me to open the connection with coca, to open my diet. Through his icaro, he was going to open my connection to the spirit of coca and its medicine.

I crawled over and sat in front of Ricardo. My vision swirled with color and increasingly bright light. As he sometimes does, Ricardo opened his song with an immediate and impressive volume. From the first syllable he was belting out magic, loud magic. My mind had already for the most part dissolved, and that icaro blew any last bits of it away. As the song continued, I felt as if I were being lifted into the air. The song was dancing in bright colors all around me, pink, orange, yellow, green, and purple. He sang in Shipibo, and in the midst of the increasingly powerful chaos, I would intermittently hear the word "coca" and catch an image of his face.

The song held me there, apparently suspended in the air, a couple of feet off the ground. I felt as if I had been lifted up by my heart.

Thoughts no longer came together; stretched beyond my mind, they could no longer reach one another. My senses were overwhelmed, suspended, hanging there; eyes open, mouth open, I could only receive. I could only experience energy, dazzling energy. This was not a matter of humbling myself. My ego had been vaporized.

After I don't know how long, he stopped and punctuated the song with some more shush shushing exhalations. He finished. My skull was an empty vessel. I could hear the people around me, but I was not sure of much else.

Ricardo then said something like, "All right Joe, let's begin."

"Begin what?" I thought. Staring blankly at him in the dark, I realized that the only thing I was clear about was that I was not ready to begin anything. I expressed this to him. I told him that I had in fact forgotten everything, including who all of these other people were, and even more confusing, why they were there with us.

Calmly, Ricardo told me in Spanish, "concéntrate." In Spanish, concentration maintains more of its connotation of collecting oneself, not just one's mind. He was asking me to concentrate my being like orange juice and he also wanted me to focus my mind. I told him that this would not be possible.

He simply repeated concéntrate. This happened at least once more. Then he changed his approach. He said he would make it easy for me. He asked me to simply take him to the person who was the most ill. "Who is the most ill?" he asked. "Who needs the most help?" He repeated, "Take me to whoever needs the most help." This, I would learn, is the path beyond confusion. Go after what is most obvious.

I could still hear a lot of groaning and rolling around. There was however one person who stood out: Russ, the sixty-something-year-old Vietnam vet who had come with our family friend Miguel. Russ seemed to be generating a virtual war zone around him. Loud vomiting, moaning, and a sense of combat caught my attention. Although we would later learn that he was having a fine time observing what he described as a galactic war between extraterrestrial forces and what sounded like mythological Hindu beings, there was, from the outside, reason for concern. Although I wasn't sure I wanted to get any closer,

I reported to Ricardo that *el amigo* Russ seemed to be doing the worst. Ricardo replied immediately, "Take me to him."

Russ is originally from Trinidad, Colorado, which during his childhood was a rural and at times violent place. When he was old enough, he joined the military and went off to Vietnam. He initially was assigned to the infantry and then transitioned over to medic work with the Dust-Off Boys (the air ambulance crew). Their job was of course to evacuate soldiers who were severely injured and dying. Russ reports that his helicopter was shot down at least seven times and additionally broke down mechanically at least another seven times. He was wounded by fragments and basically went through hell. He was exposed to some of the worst things a soldier can see, the horrors of war.

After his tour in Vietnam, he returned home an adrenaline junkie to a society that was largely unsympathetic to our veterans. He made his way out to a ranch in Colorado to try and decompress. Eventually he made his way back to school and pursued higher education. He completed a master's degree in counseling, and a master's in social work. He was able to re-integrate into society and continued with the military in the reserves. For the bulk of his career, he worked for the healthcare industry, in human resources and administration.

In the early nineties, when the Gulf War started, he began having more difficulty with post-traumatic stress disorder (PTSD) symptoms. Officially, PTSD is defined as a mental disorder that can develop after a person is exposed to a traumatic event, such as sexual assault, warfare, traffic collisions, or other threats on a person's life.[1] Symptoms include disturbing thoughts, feelings, or dreams related to the events, mental or physical distress from trauma-related cues, attempts to avoid trauma-related cues, alterations in how a person thinks and feels, and increased arousal.

During the second Gulf War, things got worse. Most of all, he was having difficulty controlling his anger. In his own words, in his workplace, "I was pretty intimidating. People were afraid of me." Russ was chronically stressed.

Russ has said, "I used to think that PTSD was a BS diagnosis until I started experiencing it myself. I saw people talking about it and my interpretation was they probably had a messed-up childhood in the first place. They're just weak individuals and can't deal with it. I got a rude awakening. It is a legitimate diagnosis."

Over the years, Russ's physical health also suffered, likely further complicated by Agent Orange exposure. After an episode of chest pain, he was diagnosed with coronary artery disease (CAD) and then eventually underwent coronary bypass surgery. He was treated medically for high blood pressure and high cholesterol. Subsequently in 1997, he had coronary stents placed to maintain blood flow in his heart. In 1998, he was also diagnosed with diabetes type II and started on medication for that as well. (History of cardiovascular disease and CAD is also a red flag when screening for participation in ayahuasca ceremony, as there exists the real possibility of heart attack or stroke during an intense experience. Before Spaceship Earth, Russ was screened by his cardiologist and passed a cardiac stress test.)

In 2003, he was officially diagnosed with PTSD. From 2003 to 2009, he underwent psychiatric treatment at the Veterans Administration (VA) for PTSD. Russ was started on fluoxetine (the SSRI Prozac) and buproprion (Wellbutrin). He also participated in individual and group therapy weekly for five months.

Vets with chronic PTSD are commonly prescribed psychoactive medications.[2] Many are also offered forms of CBT (cognitive behavioral therapy) to help them to decrease avoidance symptoms and self-blame, and to help them with acceptance, trust, and intimacy.[3] Others are treated with prolonged exposure therapy, which can be quite effective.[4] In this therapy, with the support of the therapist, patients are encouraged to recount traumatic memories over and over until their emotional reactions are diffused. Other patients improve with EMDR (eye movement desensitization and reprocessing). In this approach, participants recount disturbing memories while receiving one of several types of bilateral sensory input, e.g., side-to-side eye movements. EMDR appears to disrupt memory processing in such a way that it helps to diffuse emotional intensity associated with traumatic memories.

Russ had been on medication, he had been to psychotherapy, and he had also tried EMDR. These treatments helped to control his symptoms, however, he was not healing. By his own admission, perhaps at that time in his life, he was not really open to therapy. Russ was however interested in traditional medicine. His grandmother in New Mexico had been an herbalist, a traditional healer, and a midwife.

In 2009, Russ weaned off of his psychiatric medication in preparation for Spaceship Earth. He had previously stopped Wellbutrin and then weaned off Prozac in preparation for his plant diet. Although we have only limited information on possible drug interactions, we do know that ayahuasca can interact with certain antidepressants (the SSRIs) and related medications, potentially pushing the body into a dangerous serotonin overload syndrome. To minimize risk during treatment with the plants, Russ decided to carefully suspend his prior medications. By his own report, he did not feel much different off of the medication.

Before his first ceremony, the shamanic treatment team had an initial consultation with Russ to review his mental and physical health history. The shamans asked him why he had come. Russ says he forgot what he answered, but that he probably lied. The shamans however noticed that he was carrying a lot of stress in his shoulders and mentioned this. Russ denied it, saying that he never thought of himself as a stressed-out person. They agreed to disagree.

We decided that we would also hold his blood pressure, cholesterol, and diabetes medication for the ten-day program. We monitored his blood sugar and blood pressure throughout the experience, both of which were within normal limits while on the *vegetalista* diet.

As Ricardo and I approached him during that first Spaceship Earth ceremony, Russ was deep in his ayahuasca experience. He was looking into his body and saw dark black leeches bubbling up to the surface of his skin. They were rising up from out of his stomach and intestines. The ayahuasca was, as the Shipibos say, driving the darkness out of him. Dark leeches were oozing up and then scampering away in multiple directions. Curiously enough, Jared, another crew member seated to Russ's right, also saw these oozing creatures. This does happen in ayahuasca ceremony; sometimes multiple people share the same vision.

I sat quietly behind Ricardo, not really sure what was happening. After a bit of observation, Ricardo opened up with a relentless machine gun-style icaro that seemed to dig deeper and deeper into Russ. Once he started chanting, Russ saw that the leeches went from oozing outward to flying out of his body. As Jared witnessed, it was as if Ricardo was pulling deeper and darker leeches out of Russ's body, some with nails hanging from them. Blue sparks went flying. Jared, a bit terrified by the scene, saw electricity crackling outward. Ricardo continued his painstaking work. Russ sat up on his mat through it all, vomiting intermittently.

This shamanic cleansing went on for some time. I just sat back in the dark and tried to collect myself. The icaro continued for fifteen minutes or so and then things quieted. Russ settled down and Ricardo was satisfied.

"Joe, let's continue," he said. It was time to move on to the next person in most need of help.

Russ continued to have a very strong visionary experience that night. And for the most part his visions were inspiring. On his way outside to the toilet later on, for example, he saw all of the stars connected to one another in a light network across the night sky. When he did not return for some time, I had to retrieve him from the bathroom. He was just sitting in there, comfortable, and fascinated by the friendly, beautifully colored serpents that he saw surrounding him. In the Shipibo cosmovision, these colorful snakes often represent medicinal forms of the spirit of ayahuasca. They come to clean us energetically.

In addition to the *vegetalista* diet and the ayahuasca ceremonies, during the ten-day program, Russ was individually treated with tama-muri (*Brosimum acutifolium,* a rain-forest tree) and ajo sacha (*Mansoa alliacea,* a tropical shrub), master plants prescribed to further support his journey and his physical health, in particular, to help him with his diabetes. The entire crew of Spaceship Earth was also treated with three floral baths. Russ loved the flower baths, describing them as very cleansing and peaceful.

After his intense first ceremony, Russ continued his diet and plants and entered four more ayahuasca ceremonies as part of the program. Russ experienced significant healing during his ten days with Spaceship Earth. Here is some of what Russ had to say about his experiences with Traditional Amazonian Plant Medicine:

The first night I took the medicine, and I choose to call it medicine, it was like every synapse in my brain was firing. I can't imagine other ways that therapy would cause that. I think it helped reroute some of my patterns, my neuropatterns.

The main thing I regret about the whole PTSD thing is how I was with my kids. My daughters. . . . with my girls. I think I did a lot of damage to them. That's pretty hard to admit. Anyplace else everybody would think, "Oh he's such a nice guy, he's just so lovable, and so friendly, and so outgoing."

I learned why I do some of the things that I do, or did, with my girls. [I was too intense with them, especially about when they needed to be home.] *Don't be late.* When anybody was late in Vietnam, we had to go get them, because somebody was in trouble. That wasn't a good thing to keep thinking. I got stuck in my mind and it just carried over to my life.

During one of the ceremonies, I went and visited my kids where they live and they were asleep because it was late at night. I just looked at them and apologized for the stuff that I put them through . . . I also talked to my mother and my grandparents who are dead, just like I'm talking to you. It was powerful, very powerful.

I had some issues with my mom. [When] she was dying from cancer, she [asked] me, if it gets bad . . . will you smother me? I couldn't do it. She said that for a couple days and I felt some really big guilt after that. She was a big Kevorkian fan and that's just when he was getting in trouble. In ceremony, we talked just like we're talking now. She told me, "Son, I should've never asked you to do that. I'm sorry I did that. That was really something bad."

These experiences in the ayahuasca ceremony helped him to reconcile his past behavior and his intimate relationships, through spiritual contact with loved ones. In the mystical realms, he was able to sort through his blocks with his daughters and his mother. He was able to open his mind to greater understanding and to broader possibilities. He was able to forgive. He completed the Spaceship Earth program with flying colors. He experienced shamanic cleansing, the "re-routing of his neuropatterns," the diet, the plant treatments, and improvements in his physical health. He felt cleaner.

Months after returning home from Peru, Russ enrolled in an intensive integrative PTSD program at the Veteran's Administration (VA) in Tucson. As he says, "That integrative program was very helpful for me. I would have never gone if I had not done that work in Peru." He also joined a PTSD therapy group and he has also been helpful to others struggling with PTSD, including young veterans returning from the Middle East. He continues to live in Arizona and part-time in Colorado. Russ has not taken any psychiatric meds since Spaceship Earth. He does occasionally use marijuana medicinally.

Russ returned for three weeks of Traditional Amazonian Plant Medicine at Nihue Rao in 2014. Later that year, Russ and I presented his case in Grand Rounds at the Southwestern College of Naturopathic Medicine (SCNM). There he described this second experience quite differently. "The last trip down was a whole lot different than the first one. It was more of a physical healing," he said. During his visit to Nihue Rao (second trip to Peru), Russ took smaller doses of ayahuasca. His experiences in ceremony there were not very visual, but he still experienced significant physical purging and healing. His health continued to improve. When he left for Spaceship Earth, he weighed about 248 pounds; by the time we presented at SCNM five years later, he was down to approximately 189 pounds. His hypertension and diabetes had improved and his blood pressure and diabetes medications have been reduced. He has not had any further problems with his heart.

In response to a question at the Grand Rounds about what he gained in this process, he said, "I think forgiving myself for a lot of the stuff that I've done. For me, I think you need to forgive yourself before other people can forgive you . . . You got to be able to at least help yourself."

Russ talked about forgiveness that day, and I have come to more fully appreciate the healing power of forgiveness. Renowned Swiss psychiatrist Carl Jung remarked that forgiveness exists at the intersection between spirituality and psychology.[5] It is there helping to bridge religion and science, both a mystical process fundamental to many spiritual traditions and a psychological process vital to overcoming guilt. Forgiveness is ultimately a faculty of the psyche, or soul, and through such faculties we resonate with higher spiritual energies. Like other faculties of the psyche (e.g., gratitude, compassion, and love), forgiveness acts across the entire psychic landscape, whose terrain includes dreams as well as psychospiritual, psychological, psychiatric, psychedelic, and psychosomatic phenomena. Forgiveness is a spiritual process that heals the emotional body.

In order to forgive oneself, one starts with the mental concept and intention. You think about it and try to forgive. But nothing happens until you feel it. Once you feel it in your emotional being, in your heart and soul, then something begins to shift. You release and you accept. Forgiveness is a spiritual process that heals us emotionally. This emotional healing leads to psychological and physical improvements. As in Russ's case, ayahuasca can be helpful in this process, guiding us mystically beyond our mental prejudices and back into our hearts.

Now, what was Ricardo doing when he was unleashing his icaros on Russ that wild night in the maloka? If you ask Ricardo, he will say he was cleaning out the accumulated energies of trauma and war: from Russ's mind, his heart and soul, and from his body. Ricardo was cleaning out the unhealthy energies that he could see in his visions, chanting them out with his imagination, his medicine, and his song.

This shamanic cleansing of the energy body can also be described as a cleansing of the emotional body. Clearing this trauma energy, this dark (in Shipibo visionary terms) energy from the emotional body, often involves a visceral process, a physical purging. The emotions, as we know, are experienced physically. Emotional purging often occurs through physical processes like tears, laughter, and even vomiting and diarrhea.

Ceremonial access to a mystical state of consciousness allowed Russ to directly address his past with greater calm and understanding. Ayahuasca visions gave him the opportunity to communicate with his mother and daughters in a way that was, emotionally speaking, very real. Ayahuasca guided Russ through a process of self-forgiveness. By learning to accept himself, Russ gained access to a world beyond himself, a larger universe. He realized there were ways in which he could improve his life. There was reason to hope. Such improvements in thinking have been correlated to improvements in psychological and physical well-being, as well as improved immune function.[6,7]

Spaceship Earth was an incredible ten days and a major educational step in the fellowship. For the first time, I entered a traditional learning diet and I "assisted" Ricardo in ayahuasca ceremony. What's more, while supporting my fellow crewmembers, I got to see up close and personal how traditional treatment could impact an established Western diagnosis like PTSD. Russ's experience showed me that ayahuasca and TAPM could inspire breakthroughs even in cases of long-standing illness. Four decades after his tour in Vietnam, Russ found healing in the Amazon.

# CHAPTER 9

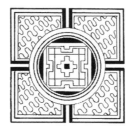

# The Emotional Body

Emotion arises at the place where mind and body meet. It is the body's reaction to your mind—or you might say, a reflection of your mind in the body.

—Eckhart Tolle

Russ's emotional healing allowed for subsequent mental and physical healing. That's how shamanic plant medicine works. It heals the mind-body by healing the emotional body.

Next we'll examine traditional treatment of PTSD and learn how shamanic medicine heals the emotional body.

After discussing Russ's case at another presentation in San Diego, I was approached by a veteran from the war in Iraq. Somewhere in Iraq, tragically, he accidentally shot and killed his close friend. He had left active duty and entered an extensive psychotherapeutic process. Through his work in therapy he was able *mentally* to accept the incident as an accident, but he was unable to forgive himself; *emotionally* he was unable to release his guilt. Eventually, he told me, he found his way to an ayahuasca ceremony. In ayahuasca ceremony he was, at last, able to clear himself emotionally and release his guilt. This is what allowed him to heal.

Healing from PTSD often requires deep emotional healing, beyond what the thinking mind can grasp. Psychedelic medicines promote deep healing in PTSD by approaching the problem holistically: psychologically, emotionally, and spiritually. From a psychological perspective, ayahuasca's effect on the brain appears to soften moral judgment and pry open closed-minded beliefs about the past.[1,2] From a shamanic perspective, this softening and expansion allow for broader acceptance and access to one's deeper emotional self. Forgiveness starts in the mind, but it is completed only in the heart.

I have often wondered how one might measure the effects of forgiveness and related spiritual healing. As mentioned, prior to Spaceship Earth, Paul Mills had joined me in Colombia for the Tukuymanta conference. Paul knew that I was headed to Iquitos with the group and suggested that I collect some anecdotal before-and-after data using a questionnaire he had worked with called the Personal Mastery Scale. On this scale, a score is calculated based on how much you agree or disagree with each of the following statements (shown below).[3]

| | Strongly Disagree | Disagree | Agree | Strongly Agree |
|---|---|---|---|---|
| 1. There is really no way I can solve some of the problems I have. | 0 ❏ | 1 ❏ | 2 ❏ | 3 ❏ |
| 2. Sometimes I feel that I am being pushed around in life. | 0 ❏ | 1 ❏ | 2 ❏ | 3 ❏ |
| 3. I have little control over the things that happen to me. | 0 ❏ | 1 ❏ | 2 ❏ | 3 ❏ |
| 4. I can do just about anything I really set my mind to do. | 0 ❏ | 1 ❏ | 2 ❏ | 3 ❏ |
| 5. I often feel helpless in dealing with the problems in life. | 0 ❏ | 1 ❏ | 2 ❏ | 3 ❏ |
| 6. What happens to me in the future mostly depends on me. | 0 ❏ | 1 ❏ | 2 ❏ | 3 ❏ |
| 7. There is little I can do to change many of the important things in my life. | 0 ❏ | 1 ❏ | 2 ❏ | 3 ❏ |

Responses to this questionnaire serve to assess one's sense of faith, in life and in oneself. Russ took this test before and after his trip with Spaceship Earth, and afterward his score improved, as did his sense of hope.

A higher Personal Mastery score has been correlated to an increased capacity to cope with stress, both psychologically and physically. Increased scores have been associated with improved functioning within the body's psychoneuroendocrine-immunologic (PNEI) network, namely in the stress response system and immune system.[4-7]

In Russ's case, profound emotional healing led to an increased sense of hope and a decrease in PTSD symptoms. His improved Personal Mastery score implied that associated improvements had also occurred in his stress response system and immune system. Improvements in his mental health and blood pressure further indicated that healing had occurred within his physical body.

Shamanic plant medicine helped to heal Russ's PTSD by healing his PNEI network (the physiologic network that links his psychology, nervous system, endocrine system, and immune system). Shamanic medicine heals the emotional body and, in concert, the mind-body.

The PNEI network is the physical manifestation of what has been called the emotional body in other traditional medical philosophies such as Ayurveda and TCM. Our emotional health, influenced by our belief system, is reflected in our emotional physiology, i.e., the functioning of this PNEI network.

PTSD is caused by emotional trauma. In PTSD, this trauma becomes imbedded in the emotional body, i.e. the PNEI network. In Russ's first ayahuasca ceremony, he saw this imbedded energy, in the form of dark black leeches, bubble up and emerge from deep within. In PTSD, deep-seated emotional trauma lurks within and disturbs multiple elements of the emotional body, causing overwhelming fear and anxiety (psychologically), an overreactive fight-or-flight response (in the nervous system), abnormal adrenaline and cortisol levels (in the hormonal/endocrine system), and out-of-control inflammation (in the immune system).[8-10]

PNEI research continues to expose the biochemical connection between the mind and body and the ways in which emotional disturbance manifests in the flesh. This mind-body research has revealed, for example, how depression impairs our ability to fight illness (from coughs and colds to cancer) and how chronic stress causes high blood pressure. The mind and body are connected. I like the way meditator and author Eckhart Tolle describes it: "Emotion arises at the place where mind and body meet." Emotion is the bridge that connects them. The PNEI network is the embodiment of this bridge.

Shipibo shamans would consider PTSD, as in the case of Russ, to be a spiritual problem caused by the accumulated energies of war and trauma. These accumulated "energies" generate dysfunction in the emotional body and its component parts. Traditionally described spiritual illness manifests as disease within the emotional body.

A core element of this emotional body is the stress response system involved in "fight or flight" responses. This stress response system is made up of the hypothalamus (in the limbic brain, central to our emotional processing), the pituitary gland (also in the limbic brain), and the adrenal glands (endocrine glands that sit on the top of the kidneys). This stress response system is referred to as the HPA axis (hypothalamus-pituitary-adrenal axis) and controls things like the production of stress hormones, namely, adrenaline and cortisol. The HPA axis is a key player in stress-related illnesses, influencing how well our bodies fight disease and control inflammation. This core element of the emotional body is the current focus of a growing body of research investigating PTSD. Emotional healing, through shamanic techniques and otherwise, heals PTSD in part by improving the function of the HPA axis (the stress response system) and other elements of the emotional body.

Psychedelic medicines continue to show great promise in the treatment of PTSD and other emotionally rooted problems. In the United States and abroad, current research into MDMA-assisted psychotherapy for PTSD has been particularly exciting.[11-14] In addition to their effects on networks like the DMN, we have learned that psychedelic medicines like MDMA and ayahuasca act directly on the limbic system, the central emotional processing center of the brain.[15-18] This key player in the emotional body also acts as a sensory integration system, integrating our experience of the outside world with what we feel within (interoception).

In 2009 during Spaceship Earth, I didn't know very much about PTSD research or about the limbic brain. But I had experienced and observed how plant medicine and spiritually oriented practices could facilitate deep emotional healing, even in difficult cases like Russ's PTSD.

Back home and in the jungle, I continued to be interested in mind-body research, but most of all, I wanted to learn more about what was going on in ceremony. I wanted to learn more about shamanism.

# CHAPTER 10

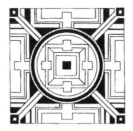

# The Beginnings of Nihue Rao Centro Espiritual

All paths are the same: they lead nowhere. . . . Does this path have a heart? If it does, the path is good; if it doesn't, it is of no use.

—Carlos Castaneda, *The Teachings of Don Juan:*
*A Yaqui Way of Knowledge*

After Spaceship Earth, I travelled to Pucallpa to continue my one-month coca diet with Rolando. I stayed there for one week in a remote tambo along the nearby lake of Yarinacocha. I then returned to the center in Iquitos to complete the last week of the process. This was my first exploration into a "learning" diet. Although the process is similar, the learning diet is distinguished from the healing diet in that the goal is to learn the medicine of the plants. The learning diet is often stricter and done for a longer period of time. Although one may also heal during a learning diet, the primary focus is to incorporate the spiritual medicine of the dieted master plant. In Ricardo's tradition, one accumulates such learning diets in order to diversify and strengthen one's medicine. This is the pathway to becoming a Shipibo *curandero* (traditional healer).

Unlike its notorious derivative cocaine (a chemical substance most often isolated in a process that involves soaking coca leaves in gasoline), the coca plant is a living being and a highly regarded medicinal plant in traditional Andean culture, across Bolivia, Peru, Ecuador, and Colombia. Coca is an extremely nutritious plant, rich in essential minerals and vitamins. The Inca (the advanced pre-Columbian civilization that had controlled much of Peru until the arrival of the Spanish conquistadors) considered coca to be the most sacred plant medicine. It is also a respected master plant in the Amazonian Shipibo tradition. I had been told that dieting coca would help me to understand its medicine and connect me to the spiritual energies of the Incas.

I was also told by the Shipibo shamans that one month would not be enough to truly connect with a master plant; they recommended a minimum of six months to initiate the connection. But I was still exploring Shipibo medicine and was not yet ready to make that kind of commitment.

I enjoyed the month-long dieting process but wasn't sure exactly what I was gaining from it. I had met other foreigners who had described a variety of incredible experiences during their learning diets. They talked about elaborate dreams and extended mental conversations with master plant spirits in the day and also during ayahuasca visions. I did not have that kind of experience. For me the learning diet was a subtle process.

On the last night of my month-long coca diet, in ayahuasca ceremony, I did have brief visions of spirits in traditional Incan dress. Perhaps this was just my imagination or projection, or maybe this was the connection I was looking for. I could not be sure. Either way, this vision encouraged me to diet further.

While I was still completing my diet in Peru, Miguel went back to Phoenix. He had had his own transformational experience during Spaceship Earth. In particular, he saw the cycle of violence in his family's past and how this had impacted his own family. Back in Arizona, he shared these experiences with my parents who were still quite doubtful about my involvement in the Amazon. He also told my father about Russ's progress. My father had noted a change in Miguel and was quite curious about the shifts that had occurred in Russ.

At the end of my diet, I returned to the United States, back to the lab and to part-time work as a doctor. Soon after, I had a chance to discuss my Spaceship Earth experiences with my father. We spoke on the phone for twenty minutes or so. In particular, he wanted to know about what had happened to Miguel and Russ in ceremony. I shared some of the mysterious details. That phone conversation was the only time I ever really got the chance to speak with my father as a medical colleague.

A couple of months later, in June of 2009, my dad passed away. Although there was no autopsy or hospital intervention, it appears he died of a heart attack. In the fall, I moved home to Arizona to help settle my father's affairs and to go through the grieving process with my family.

As time went on, I applied for a medical license in Arizona and began working as a *per diem* physician in Phoenix. As a *per diem* physician, I could take short-term work for two to three months at a time. This gave me the time and flexibility I needed to explore Amazonian plant medicine further.

## Ayahuasca Tourism

It was around that time that I began to learn more about the problems that plague ayahuasca tourism. Growing numbers of visitors coming to experience *la medicina* have brought an economic boon to places like Iquitos. This new economy has given rise to many new healing centers and, inevitably, to an increasing number of ayahuasca charlatans. Tales of extraordinary experiences have spread across the Internet and contribute to an already confused and overly romanticized view of traditional ayahuasca culture, and at the same time many economically frustrated South Americans are seizing the opportunity to take advantage of naïve foreign adventurers.

There has always been a dark side to ayahuasca shamanism. As in most fields, this dark side is about power and the manipulation of others. Many people have been misled by phony shamans. Others have fallen under the spell of those with darker intentions. In particular, women have been taken advantage of and abused by some Amazonian shamans. The local Peruvians are well aware of this problem. However, foreigners are not so well-informed. Many vulnerable women, especially those seeking healing for sexual abuse, are particularly susceptible to sexual predators. There have been a number of cases of sexual molestation and rape, within and connected to ayahuasca ceremony.

For this reason, I always caution travelers to be very careful about whom they drink ayahuasca with. The best way to find a trustworthy shaman is through a trusted personal recommendation. When in Peru, do as the Peruvians. Approach shamanic culture cautiously and learn as much as you can about the reputation and integrity of the shaman you are interested in working with.

I was, of course, disappointed to hear about these unethical and damaging behaviors. But I also saw, again and again, the potential for profound healing with ayahuasca and associated plant medicines. Over the years, I explored a number of ayahuasca traditions. I entered ceremonies with an indigenous Kamsá shaman from Colombia, an Ashaninka shaman from Peru, and a mestizo shaman from the Iquitos area. In these experiences, I met several skilled and ethical healers. Ultimately though, I found myself most interested in the indigenous Shipibo tradition. In some of the other traditions I observed, the shaman facilitated the group experience without getting involved in individual healings. As a physician, I was more interested in the kind of one-on-one shamanic doctoring practiced in Shipibo ceremony. Furthermore, the Shipibo language is still very much alive and the tradition seemed more connected to its pre-Columbian roots.

After a couple more journeys to South America, I returned to Iquitos in July of 2010 to work with Ricardo Amaringo. I had personally experienced the impact of his powerful icaros and had witnessed their effects on others like Russ. Ricardo had impressed me with his sensitivity to my field of consciousness. When he sang to me, he appeared to track my mind's focus. Wherever I placed my attention, he would follow. If, for example, I focused on the area over my right shoulder, he would perk up and look over my right shoulder. If I focused on my stomach, he would direct his song there. Ricardo is also someone who respects the importance of protecting women during vulnerable healing experiences. On several occasions, we had discussed the importance of creating a safe ceremonial environment for women.

During that stay, I completed another four-week learning coca diet under Ricardo. My primary intention was to gain some clarity about my future with traditional Amazonian medicine. I was in part concerned that my journeys to the Amazon were becoming a distraction from continuing forward in my medical career. To be honest, I was also a little embarrassed to be so interested in a spiritual practice that involved a mind-altering substance. I was truly torn. In South America, ayahuasca is regarded as an important component of traditional Amazonian treatment, and I had been very impressed by the outcomes that I observed. In North American culture, however, ayahuasca was regarded as a "New Age" hallucinogenic drug, something for hippies and free spirits, perhaps, but not for serious doctors.

I asked Ricardo to try and help me understand why I was still coming down to the Amazon to drink ayahuasca. Ricardo told me that he could not directly say, but that he would beg the spirits to explain it to me.

My mind battled it, but deep inside, in my heart, I knew that ayahuasca shamanism had the power to heal in a way that I had never seen before. I had felt it. It was as real to me as anything I had learned in medical school.

In one of my most significant ayahuasca visions during that diet, I saw myself sitting in a magical office somewhere in the Amazon forest. The office itself was a simple square wooden building with a desk and chair. However, inside, every surface—the walls, the furniture, the ceiling, and floor—all glowed in brilliant orange, yellow, and white. In those colors, Shipibo plant medicine designs scrolled across everything in the room. These bold patterns flowed with a living vibrancy and a palpable intelligence, plant intelligence. I sat on the floor as the energies flowed all around me, above and below. As

I looked around the room, I saw that there were many books and papers stacked on the desk's magical surface and across the luminous floor. I got the feeling that it was a glimpse into a possible future. It was a vision about academic study in the jungle, within the tradition.

In the following days, Ricardo told me of his interest in starting his own career as a maestro. After years of training and apprenticeship, he felt ready to strike out on his own. During that visit in 2010, I met fellow *pasajeros* Cvita Mamic from Alberta, Canada and her then-boyfriend (now husband) Markus Drassl from South Tyrol, Italy. They had both been dieting for personal healing for several months at the center and had spent a lot of time with Ricardo. They, like me, were fans of his medicine. Ricardo had also shared his plans with another couple, my friends Soi Bari and Flor. With Ricardo's invitation, we decided to work with him to realize his dream of starting a new healing center.

This would be a place where the safety of the *pasajeros*, especially women, would be prioritized. He had already identified a potential location and wanted to know if we would invest in this idea and help him to administer the center. As soon as I heard Ricardo's proposal, my doubts about life direction cleared. My work with Spaceship Earth had been some of the most rewarding work I had ever been a part of. I wanted to be a part of more of that kind of healing, deep spiritual healing. I knew immediately that I wanted to be part of the new center.

## Nihue Rao is Born

A few days later, we all travelled out to see the empty property. In total, it was about 19 acres. A large central section had been cleared for charcoal production and yucca farming. Together, during that visit, we decided to buy it. Ricardo was particularly interested in the property as it was home to a rare grove of *nihue rao* trees, sacred in the Shipibo tradition. For just six hundred dollars, I became one of the initial investors in what would eventually become the healing center Nihue Rao Centro Espiritual. The name is meant to capture the Shipibo and mestizo elements of our staff's culture. Nihue Rao is the name of the sacred tree in Shipibo. (*Nihue* means breath or wind or air; *Rao* means medicine as in plant medicine.) We kept the words *Centro Espiritual* in Spanish to honor the mestizo culture that predominates in Peru and much of Latin America.

The next day or so, the original six of us went in to town to take care of the paperwork. I continued my dieting and completed the month, gaining a bit more experience and insight into Shipibo shamanism. During one memorable ceremony, I witnessed the icaro at work. The tea was having a rather mild effect on me that night and I had more or less given up on having visions. I lay back to rest, but as I turned my head on the pillow, I noticed that one of the shamans was singing to someone nearby. I glanced over and noticed that the *pasajero* was lying on his back, the shaman seated to his side. As I looked and listened, I saw the shaman's icaro take form. The icaro became a swirling, glowing vortex extending from his mouth to the participant's abdomen. Between them, this energy vortex undulated with the melody of the song. The icaro's "edges" vibrated in such a way that they matched the frequency of the participant's energy body. This energy body appeared as a complex arrangement of vibrating, illuminated beads. The vortex targeted the abdomen, and there, its energies merged with the vibrating beads of the body in order to open a tunnel, an energetic scope into the abdomen.

Off to one side of the shaman, looking into this swirling tunnel, I could see the participant's internal organs. Through the icaro, the shaman was scanning his body. Briefly, I could see his organs as I had seen them during surgery in the operating room. The song continued, but the vortex was then turned away from me. The vision faded.

The next day I told Ricardo what I had seen. He simply looked at me and said, "*Así es*" (that's how it is) and confirmed that I was beginning to learn something.

Once my coca diet was complete, I returned to Arizona. Things shifted among the original partners, and our team dwindled down to just Ricardo, Cvita, and me. We had hoped for a larger team to share the workload, but that wasn't to be. At that point, I did not know

Cvita very well, but she has turned out to be a true sister to me. She is a beautiful and brilliant healer/artist and a tough businesswoman. She had had significant management experience and had also been successful as a visual artist. The three of us combined our respective skills and experience in shamanism, management, art, allopathic medicine, and spiritual healing to build the new center.

In December of 2010, Cvita and I began sending money down to Ricardo as he supervised the early construction of Nihue Rao. Although it seemed like a wild gamble, Ricardo and the team showed themselves to be responsible and committed to the success of the project. Early construction was completed out in the jungle without power tools or, for that matter, electricity. Ricardo was aided by our Portuguese friend Paolo and his family, our Peruvian friends Tito and Hugo, and a whole crew of hardworking laborers. The maloka was nearly done by New Year's, and in the early spring of 2011, Nihue Rao opened to receive our first guests.

# CHAPTER 11

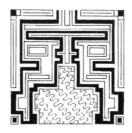

# The Placebo Effect and Unexplainable Chronic Cough

*There is no substitute for self-love.*

—anonymous

In April of 2011, I arrived at the center ready to work. Those early days at Nihue Rao were pretty tough, living conditions were rough, and business was up and down. Ricardo's reputation as a healer helped to keep us afloat. *Pasajeros* trickled in.

By the summer of 2011, we had a team of three Shipibo shamans working in the ceremony. Ricardo was our lead shaman and he was assisted by Julian Arevalo, who was in his late thirties. We were also joined by the established elder, Julian's mother, Olivia Arevalo who was at that time probably in her seventies. Olivia is well known in the shamanic community and has practiced Shipibo shamanism since her youth. By the time she came to Nihue Rao, she had already been working with foreigners at other nearby healing centers.

I find Olivia's icaros particularly beautiful and very hypnotic. In her song, I hear a series of intricately moving parts. Her icaros, like the visions, are a kaleidoscope of moving energies. Julian, her son, is a natural talent raised in the tradition. Perhaps this was why he was a bit less disciplined. Nonetheless, he is very gifted in shamanic vision and healing power, and his icaros helped us to build Nihue Rao's reputation.

One of my jobs at Nihue Rao was to assist in ceremony by helping people to the bathroom or bringing them up to the shamans for their individualized healing. In the early days, Cvita and I would do this work. From time to time, Ricardo would send me over to try and help soothe someone who was having a hard time. I would mostly just sit with them; sometimes I would experiment with a shush shushing whistle to calm them. Sometimes I would pray for them. I learned that with the proper intention I could also use mapacho smoke to help calm them.

Ricardo would also ask me on occasion to blow Agua de Florida (an alcohol-based perfume) on *pasajeros* overwhelmed by the effect. The scent of the Agua de Florida can be used to help bring someone to their senses. That was how the early unofficial apprenticeship worked. I was to stay alert to the ceremony and follow Ricardo's cues. I would sometimes drink ayahuasca, but for the most part I had to be careful not to overdo it.

After ceremonies, in the morning, we would all sit together and review the night's experiences, adjust treatments, and prepare for the next ceremony. These debriefings are similar to daily hospital rounds, during which the medical team reviews the night's events. The morning conversation was also a time to review some of my own experiences with the shamans. Julian has a particular gift for "third eye" vision, and on a few occasions he surprised me with his ability to read my mind.

# A Little White Magic

One morning I asked him about something I had heard him singing to me the night before. He sings in Shipibo but once in a while he'll use a little Spanish. I had heard him chant the word *libro*. I don't think they have a word for book in Shipibo and so they use the Spanish term *libro*. When I heard this word during the chant, my first reaction was, "These superstitious shamans, he probably wants me to stop reading a certain book." Sometimes they are suspicious of the energies associated with certain books.

I asked him why he was singing to me about a *libro*.

Julian replied, "You're reading that book right now, aren't you?"

"Yes, I am reading a book," I told him.

"Well, that's fascinating, really fascinating. What is that about?" he said.

"It's about the placebo effect," I told him.

"That's a white magic (*magia blanca*), very interesting," Julian said.

That was a nice idea, the placebo effect as a white magic. I had been reading *The Placebo Effect*, a book that presents varied opinions on the role of placebo in modern medicine. I particularly liked the chapter by Dr. Howard Brody "The Doctor as Therapeutic Agent: A Placebo Effect Research Agenda."[1] Dr. Brody writes:

Positive placebo response is most likely to occur when the meaning attached to that illness experienced by the patient is altered in a positive direction. Meaning in turn consists of at least three general components: providing an understandable and satisfying explanation of the illness to the person; demonstrating care and concern; and holding out an enhanced promise of mastery or control over the symptoms.

That is the white magic of a placebo, very useful in any medical tradition. The meaning we attach to illness is often a hot topic during post-ceremony conversations. I often translated during these meetings. Afterwards Ricardo would sometimes ask me to speak further with our guests to follow up with them about their experience. Through further conversation and processing, we would try to determine how best to help them. We needed to learn about the meaning they had attached to their illness. As a medical doctor, I would also review our guests' medical histories. Although not all of the Amazonian healing centers have a physician available to review a person's medical history, many of the centers recognize the crucial importance of reviewing a client's relevant medical history. Clients on any allopathic maintenance medications, clients with a history of severe mental illness or emotional disturbance, clients who have suffered severe trauma—all these must be handled with great skill and sensitivity. And sometimes it is simply too dangerous for a given individual to work with the sacred plants.

One particularly memorable visitor from those early days was a woman named Colleen. She had been struggling with a chronic dry cough for years.

Colleen had been involved in an international nonprofit organization that was providing free surgeries to underserved Peruvians. After one of their medical brigades, one of her colleagues had come to visit our center. In one of her ayahuasca ceremonies in the visions, this woman clearly saw Colleen sitting next to her in the maloka. It was such a strong vision that she felt compelled to share it with Colleen and encouraged her to visit us.

Colleen wanted to come, but she could only get away for one night. Nihue Rao does not normally take people for just one ceremony, first of all, because serious treatment involves an extended plant diet, and second, because Ricardo and the shamans don't want to work with people who simply want to dabble in the medicine. These shamans are highly trained individuals who prefer to work with people who are committed enough to the experience to stick around for a week or more. But Colleen was a special case. She had a very busy schedule and she was helping Peruvian children. We decided to accommodate her for just the one night.

Colleen arrived in Iquitos by plane and then took the ninety-minute all terrain mototaxi ride out to Nihue Rao Centro Espiritual. The latter sixty minutes of that journey takes you down a rather bumpy, unpaved, and potentially muddy road. Nihue Rao sits adjacent to the expansive Allpahuayo Mishana National Reserve. On your way there, initially, you pass a rural community known as Zungarococha. The road then cruises you past the Nanay River and through a number of small communities, including the neighboring jungle village of Llanchama. Colleen's mototaxi brought her through the center's forested entrance. She then stepped down onto the white, sandy soil. She was quickly settled into her rustic room and then brought over to the medicine house to take her plant vomitive. Although it was just for one night, she wanted to go the extra mile to maximize her experience.

We then sat together and reviewed her intentions for her brief time with us and discussed her medical and personal history. Colleen's cough was very uncomfortable, interrupting her speech and other activities, and sometimes made it difficult for her to sleep. Her colleague confirmed that when she shared a room with Colleen, she heard her coughing all night. Chronic cough can have many causes.[2,3] Back home, Colleen's primary doctor had done an initial workup and ruled out infection. Her medical team then explored the possibility of underlying asthma, allergy, or esophageal reflux. No clear diagnosis was determined. She was then sent to a pulmonologist for further evaluation, which included pulmonary function testing and CT (computerized tomography) scans.

After an extensive workup, Colleen's doctors determined that she suffered from Idiopathic Chronic Cough. This is the doctor's way of saying we don't know why she has a chronic cough (idiopathic is taken from the Greek and means something like "a disease of its own kind").

Colleen is a well-educated woman and had for many years worked diligently and successfully in corporate America. In the last few years, she had decided to take a break from the corporate world to use her skills for something more meaningful. She had been focusing her attention on these much-needed medical brigades. This turned out to be the right move for her. Years later, she continues to be very passionate and happy about her work with the nonprofit.

Colleen explained that in her broad search to find help for her cough, she had gone to see a spiritual healer in the United States, some kind of seer. The seer told her that the medical doctors would not be able to help her with this cough because it was a symptom of a spiritual wound. She would need the help of someone who could heal spiritual illness.

Colleen told me that she did not think that her cough originated from her lungs, she thought that it started somewhere in her solar plexus, in the area of the third chakra as described in Hindu metaphysics. That is where she *felt* it originating. She began to tell me the story of her childhood. Her parents had a troubled marriage (which subsequently resulted in a divorce) and were not always present for her. Consequently, she had had to take on the added responsibility of helping to raise her younger siblings. She missed out on a lot of her childhood. In short, she experienced a real lack of love and support at the beginning of her life.

She grew up and eventually met a man and fell in love. She was happy to leave her family's house and in many ways everything seemed much better. She was excited about becoming a committed and loyal wife. She dedicated herself to her husband for over twenty years. Then, the year before her visit to Nihue Rao, she found out that he had been cheating on her. It appears that he had been cheating with multiple partners and that this had been going on for years. She was blindsided by this revelation. She was devastated both by the deceit and by her own inability to see what had been going on. She had always tried to do the right thing. She had thought that everything was fine.

I could see that there was a lot of dissonance in her life.

I took her over to Julian and Olivia to discuss her case further and to make a plan for the ceremony. They were sitting out in front of their small house on the property. I explained to them that she had only one night because she was busy helping Peruvians, but that we were really hoping to make a difference in her case. I explained the history of her cough and the recent developments of her personal life.

Olivia prefers not to speak too much in Spanish, but she listened and then explained to Julian in Shipibo. Julian translated back to us that her cough was indeed coming from her solar plexus because that was where she was storing her *pena*, as we say in Spanish, her grief and her shame. Whether or not she was doing this consciously, it was there. As I translated to Colleen, her face softened. She had been heard, and now I could see that she was curious to hear more. Olivia said that we needed to clean her *pena* from her solar plexus. The plan was to approach this energy shamanically in ayahuasca ceremony.

After we spoke with the shamans, I walked Colleen over to the maloka to discuss the ceremony further. Before someone's first time, it is important to review the possible "symptoms" of the ayahuasca experience. It is not uncommon to experience nausea, vomiting, diarrhea, excessive fatigue and weakness, body temperature disturbances, intense sweating, flowing tears, frequent yawning, involuntary body movements, and/or physical pain. These experiences vary from person to person and from ceremony to ceremony. As much as possible, I tried to prepare participants for these potential reactions, as they can be alarming. Yet, no matter how much you orient people, at least a few will be convinced that they have been temporarily poisoned. The reality is that the ayahuasca experience is hard work. There is no way around this work. The experience is different every time, sometimes very pleasant, other times more difficult. We must always be ready to put in some work.

Later that evening, we headed into ceremony. Colleen's intention was to heal her spiritual wound. She hoped to gain greater understanding and heal her cough. I poured her a small amount of ayahuasca. It was her first time and I wanted to be careful. I let her know that after an hour or so I would check on her. Time passed and the shamans began singing icaros. After about an hour, I went to see how she was doing.

She said, "Uh, I don't know, I'm not sure if I feel anything."

I brought her over to the ayahuasca and gave her a bit more. I encouraged her to focus on her intention and to ask for help from the ayahuasca. The shamans had been singing icaros to the maloka. Soon after, I started bringing the *pasajeros* up for their individualized songs. At some point, it seemed like the right moment to bring Colleen up to Olivia. I walked across the dark maloka with my red flashlight, careful to minimize its shine.

"Colleen, how are you doing?" I whispered.

The Placebo Effect and Unexplainable Chronic Cough       99

"You know, I feel a little altered," she replied. She was not having a major experience, but she was showing some signs of the *mareación*. Once on her feet, she was a little unsteady. I quietly walked her over to sit down on the mat in front of Olivia, bucket in hand, just in case. I let Olivia know that this was the woman we had spoken with earlier, the one with the *pena* in her solar plexus. Then they just sat across from each other in silence for some time. Olivia was looking at her, in her shamanic visions, studying her to make a plan for the song. Olivia was looking into her energy body, to see what needed to be cleaned. This is the first step for the *ayahuasquera/o*, to look and see what the ayahuasca reveals.

I sat down nearby to watch. After some moments, Olivia opened up with her song, sweet and mystical. Colleen sat quietly in the dark listening to the high-pitched melodic vibrations of the icaro. Then, about 30 seconds into the chant, Colleen took a deep breath and suddenly burst into sobbing tears. She wept in catharsis. After a few minutes, spastic crying had her diaphragm heaving and she began to vomit. I have seen a lot of vomiting and this was some heavy duty vomiting. And crying. Then her cough started up, hacking, then coughing, vomiting and coughing. I don't know how long Olivia sang to her, maybe for fifteen or twenty minutes. Eventually Colleen's cough trailed off and Olivia finished singing. I walked over to help her back to her spot.

"How was that, Colleen?" I said.

"Whoa, that was amazing. It was like she was inside of me and I was inside of her and it was so beautiful," she whispered. (She later told me that during the song Olivia had appeared to her as a bluebird singing, perched on her heart.)

I walked her back to her mat. After she went through the cleaning process with Olivia, she entered a new phase of her ayahuasca experience. She began to have a series of visions and then a number of realizations. First, all of her ancestors from beyond her parents came to her. They surrounded her and gave her all of the love that her parents had not able to give her when she was growing up. She was overwhelmed with this love. Then, she reported, she felt herself opening to a new level of self-love and acceptance. She had not previously believed that her family had loved her in that way. In the visions her ancestors told her, "We love you unconditionally. It's okay to love yourself all the way. You don't need to settle for second best."

After this experience being surrounded with love, she saw a vision of her husband and started focusing on his sexual addiction. She saw him as a young child curled up on the floor with a man standing over him. Although the details were not clear, she received the message that he had been abused as a child. This resonated with her and through this understanding she was able to find a new compassion for him. She knew that she did not want to stay with him, but this helped her to understand the nature of his secretive behavior.

After the ceremony, I asked her about her experience. She said that when she was vomiting, she saw orange and red rocks shooting out of her mouth. She said there was no bile, no stomach fluid, only orange and red rocks. I told Julian about what she described. He replied, "Of course, that wasn't from her stomach, it wasn't something bad she ate, that was from her life, from the story of her life, that was the energy that was in there." For some reason, the energy appeared as orange and red rocks, somehow petrified and calcified over the years.

She reported feeling better after the ceremony. She was not sure what to do about the visionary revelation concerning her husband. Sometimes the ayahuasca speaks through metaphor, describing patterns of energy exchange. Other times the information revealed is more concrete. It takes time to discern the difference.

In the morning, after some more conversation, it was time for Colleen to head out on her way.

The shamans wanted to have more time with her to make more progress, but this was not possible.

When I followed up with Colleen a couple of months later, she still had a little bit of the cough. But in all of her adventures in healthcare, she said, that one night had given her the most significant relief she had felt in years. She had also started her divorce process. She told me that she felt like the cough would resolve completely once the divorce was finalized.

She also told me, "When it's too much, when I can't take it anymore, I just remember. I just sit myself down in front of Olivia again in my head and I'm right there with her and it's just, all of a sudden, I can do it again." A song can reframe the story of your life and help you to transform your pain into useful lessons.

That was five years ago. I recently checked in on her, five years later, to review her progress. Her cough is gone. It progressively improved as she suspected it would, as she worked through the divorce process. Along the way she learned that her ex-husband, in addition to the cheating, had maintained a separate family for years. But she was not derailed by this revelation.

Somewhere along the way, earlier in life, Colleen had closed her mind to her feelings. A lack of love, self-love, and unreleased pain were left unattended in her being. This left blind spots in her emotional consciousness, which clouded her awareness. Spiritual healing helped Colleen cleanse her grief, find self-love, and revitalize her emotional body. This gave her the start she needed to walk down a longer road of healing. Colleen is now physically healthier, mentally more aware, and she loves herself more fully.

## So Doctor, What "Actually" Happened Here?

In treating any medical condition, including chronic cough, the hope is to address the underlying cause. In Colleen's case, all suspected medical causes were ruled out. She perceived ongoing discomfort in the region of her solar plexus, and the shaman linked that feeling to emotional stagnation and the dissonance between her conscious awareness and her subconscious emotional experience. As I once heard a Native American healer say, "The heart does not close. The mind closes to the heart, one can turn the mental switches off to one's feelings, but the heart remains open and continues to feel." The heart continues to feel what is around us, whether or not we are consciously aware.

This emotional stagnation in Colleen's body and this dissonance between mind and feeling appear to have been the underlying cause of her cough, her spiritual wound. This was addressed shamanically through healing song under the influence of ayahuasca. Again, this process included further mystical revelations pertinent to her healing process. Disturbances in the emotional body are often connected to what have traditionally been described as energetic disturbances. In Colleen's case, this disturbance could be traced to the third chakra, an energetic center in the body traditionally associated with self-esteem.

In Colleen's case, a positive placebo response was achieved in the sense that the meaning attached to her cough was altered in a positive direction. Through her idiopathic cough, her soul, you might say, was crying out to her. Her cough eventually drew her attention to what she had for some time neglected to notice. Ultimately, she needed to learn how to love herself more fully. This love would help her to overcome the self-neglect she had grown accustomed to. In order to heal, she would need to open her mind to her feelings. Through just one ayahuasca treatment, she was able to find an understandable and satisfying explanation of her illness. With proper care and concern, she was able to find mastery over her symptoms.

Doctors would characterize this sort of chronic cough as a form of psychosomatic illness, a physical illness or other condition caused or aggravated by a mental factor such as internal conflict or stress. True to its name, psychosomatic illness is often rooted in the psyche (soul). Psychosomatic symptoms are one way in which the psyche can alert the conscious mind to a deeper problem. Healthcare providers should remember this possibility as they try to determine the root of so-called idiopathic and psychosomatic illnesses. If a health problem is spiritual in nature, i.e., if it is a soul sickness, then it may require spiritual treatment.

The emotional body as I describe it includes the PNEI network—the brain's limbic system, the autonomic nervous system, which controls subconscious body functioning (like breathing and digestion), the endocrine system, and the immune system. The autonomic nervous system, which controls breathing, is wired directly into the emotional processing center of the brain (the limbic system). In the case of psychosomatic cough (in which other causes have been ruled out), scientific researchers have identified at least two disturbances in the PNEI network that can be linked to emotional problems. First, the vagus nerve (one of the autonomic nerve that controls breathing) becomes hypersensitive.[4] This hypersensitive vagus nerve generates trigger-happy coughing, even in the absence of any significant irritant or airway blockage. In other words, the person coughs when it is not physically necessary. Secondly, there is *neurogenic* inflammation, abnormal inflammation in the airways generated by the nervous system and brain.[5] This neurogenic inflammation occurs in the absence of any apparent physical wound or injury. Emotional disturbances can generate neurogenic inflammation in the PNEI network.

Neurogenic inflammation is one of the ways that the emotional body declares itself. This form of inflammation could be described as a potential indication of a spiritual wound, or at the very least, a sign of an emotional problem. Although Western doctors are trying to develop medications to address various forms of neurogenic inflammation, such treatment will not likely address underlying emotional problems.

Neurogenic inflammation is currently gaining more and more attention, as it appears to be involved in a wide range of health problems (which in some cases are psychosomatic in nature), including asthma, allergic rhinitis, chronic cough, psoriasis, migraine headaches, and fibromyalgia.[6]

For years, Colleen's emotional body was crying out to her through vagus nerve hypersensitivity and neurogenic inflammation in her lungs. These are the dynamic physiologic processes that reflected the energetic disturbances in her emotional body. In ayahuasca ceremony, these emotionally derived energetic disturbances were able to be addressed, opening the door for deeper healing.

# CHAPTER 12

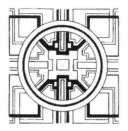

# Healing Hidden Trauma

That is the way it is with a wound. The wound begins to close in on itself, to protect what is hurting so much. And once it is closed, you no longer see what is underneath, what started the pain.

—Amy Tan, *The Joy Luck Club*

Deeper healing takes time. As most health problems do not develop overnight, most are not cured overnight. In Colleen's case, however, that one night was very impactful and set her on a longer road to profound healing. That road took her through five tough years, during which she divorced and underwent many personal changes. Over the months and years, her cough improved and then eventually resolved. Spiritual healing involves raising your consciousness and changing the way you live. Changing the way one lives takes time. This is why the work that goes on after ceremony is so important.

In those early days at the center, during our first year, our intensive work in the jungle chugged along. We were a new business struggling to become self-sustaining. We started with only a few buildings (the maloka, four bathrooms, one shower, quarters for the workers, an office, and the kitchen) and almost no furniture. Little by little we started building beds and tables and couches and things. For some time, we were more or less broke, but we were happy. Living in the jungle was full of excitement and beauty. Things are simpler when you are at the mercy of the elements, in our case, rain, mud, floods, and tropical sunshine.

Our Peruvian employees, mostly local villagers, often helped to lighten the mood. In fact, generally speaking, most of them are at all times on the verge of explosive laughter; hooting, hollering, knee-slapping laughter. Nature, community, and spirit are on their side. Out in the jungle, the existential crises that trouble the materialist world seem kind of boring. They have frustrations, disappointments, and economic concerns, but in general, they consciously choose happiness over misery.

Initially I stayed at Nihue Rao for about four months at a time. I would head home to Arizona and work as a *per diem* physician, sending down what money I could. Cvita and I both continued to invest in the center. We developed our website and did what we could to draw clients. Ricardo was well known from his work at the other center and this helped a great deal. Chris Kilham, medicine hunter, educator, and author, and his wife Zoe Helene, artist, cultural activist, and journalist, as well as others helped to promote us through media outlets on the Internet. Thanks to Zoe, we also gained the support of journalist Amber Lyon and her impressive website reset.me. Over time, we reinvested our profits back into the business, and with the help of a number of ingenious Peruvians, bit by bit, we improved the infrastructure of the center.

At Nihue Rao there are four ayahuasca ceremonies per week. This is a pretty intense schedule. Ricardo insisted that we maintain this schedule in order to adequately help those who come from so far away. Over the first year, I was gaining experience, but still not sure whether or not I myself wanted to undergo formal training to become an *ayahuasquero*. Ricardo, on the other hand, was very sure that he wanted both of his business partners, both Cvita and me, to train and learn under him.

Ricardo's master only rarely gave him any explicit guidance, as *aya-huasqueros* generally believe that most of the learning happens intuitively and through practice. For the most part, we were trained in that tradition. Ricardo did however throw us a few pearls of wisdom here and there as we worked through the ceremonies.

As we went along, he continued to push me to help the *pasajeros* through their journeys. By the time I had started working at Nihue Rao, I had completed two month-long coca diets, one during Spaceship Earth and one during the initial purchase of the Nihue Rao property. These diets, although short by Ricardo's standards, were focused on learning shamanism, although in the Shipibo tradition healing and learning ultimately occur together. In those early days at Nihue Rao, I dieted an additional third month with coca. My experiences with coca continued to be subtle. Even in subtlety though, the plant managed to inspire me through our difficult work.

One ceremony night, for example, I was again visited by Incan spirits in my visions. That day I was worn out from late nights in ceremony and long days heading into town to use the Internet. Those long days were made even longer when I needed to (once again) engage the tired Peruvian bureaucracy. In that vision, I saw myself, exhausted, sitting in front of a government desk filling out some papers. Just as it seemed I would succumb to the fatigue and give up, four Incan spirits, glowing in traditional dress, boldly colored caps and ponchos, came up behind me and filled me with their light. They lifted me up to my feet and gave me the energy I needed to continue.

The next morning, I headed back into town with Ricardo. After a long night of ceremony, he had fallen asleep as we patiently waited for our number to be called at the bank. I woke him up to tell him what had happened to me the night before. I told Ricardo that it seemed as if our work was not just about partnering with each other and with Cvita but also about partnering with plant spirits. Ricardo smiled and said something like, "*Son cosas increíbles, muy difícil de creer*" (these are incredible things, very difficult to believe), "*así es la dieta*" (that is how the diet is). Little by little, I learned about working with plant spirits.

At Nihue Rao, I learned a lot about traditional healing from the plants and from Ricardo, but perhaps I learned the most from our *pasajeros*. I learned a great deal from one particular *pasajera,* Maria, and her extended healing process. She helped me to understand how childhood emotional trauma can affect adult health.

In December 2012, Maria arrived. She had heard about us through friends and had been to another center back in 2010 or thereabouts. She was in her mid-thirties and had been struggling with her health for years. She was depressed, fatigued, struggling with her weight, and in chronic pain. Despite her ailments, she had managed to be a positive person, leading and organizing a number of community projects and working diligently on her music career as a singer/songwriter.

When she arrived to the center, she was planning to stay for one month, which Ricardo believed would be sufficient time to see some improvement in her condition. In addition to her depression and fatigue, she also reported "serious food allergies." "No matter what I eat, I either get really tired and fall asleep or get skin rashes. No matter what, even if I eat fish, it makes me sick. Vegetables . . . it doesn't matter what it is," she said.

Her depression was further complicated by chronic pain. Initially, the problem was in her left knee. She had had two prior knee surgeries, ten years apart, both for torn cartilage. She recovered well after the first surgery, but after the second injury and surgery, she struggled with intermittent pain and limited range of motion. Her knee problem gave rise to a back problem. She developed chronic sciatica in her right leg and lower back and was diagnosed with a bulging disk in her lumbar spine. She had been treated with steroid spinal injections twice but had not improved.

With her worsening back and knee problems, her overall mobility was increasingly limited. "It was like my body was hardening or solidifying," she recalled. "I also couldn't lose weight. It didn't matter what I ate . . . I think I had severe inflammation," she stated.

She was frustrated with her medical care. Her primary care physician had told her that sometimes these problems are "all in your head" and that he didn't have any further treatment options for her. She then saw another doctor. This doctor was more seriously concerned about her psychological state. She told Maria that she had screened positive for depression, and that she should seek treatment. Maria admits that at that time she was too angry to consider treatment. She refused psychotherapy and never took antidepressant medication.

She did however continue to look for other forms of help. She eventually found a structural medicine practitioner/physical therapist who was able to reach her at a more personal level. "She got me to walk again, but we hit a point with the work where she couldn't get me any further," said Maria. This therapist advised her that her problems were of an emotional nature. She suggested to Maria that she would not improve until her emotional issues were addressed. Maria had been through a lot of emotional abuse as a child and adolescent and knew she had a lot of healing work to do, but she had never really connected that with her physical problems.

Through her community in the Pacific Northwest, Maria had heard about ayahuasca and Traditional Amazonian Plant Medicine. In 2010, she travelled to Iquitos for a ten-day experience. In those ten days, she dieted several plants, although she does not remember which ones. Her first experience with ayahuasca and Amazonian plant medicine was very difficult and involved a lot of physical pain, but she did feel that the treatment shifted things in her life, and she felt more focused. In her own words, "It got me to start asking for what I needed in my relationships and voicing issues I was having . . . I was so used to being in a traumatized state I wasn't able to actually voice or identify my feelings . . . At some point it would become overwhelming. I'd either check out of the friendship or continue to kind of take the unbalanced relationship for what it was. It [the healing] started to get me to call some friends out for flaking out on things they agreed to. I shared my anger and frustration and all that kind of stuff." She felt that the first diet had helped her to address relationships and sparked more free and sincere expression. She was then able to tell people, "This isn't good enough for me, I have to tell you."

Afterward, however, she continued to struggle with back pain, which was worse after walking for long distances. She felt she was too young to be suffering in this way. Maria decided that she wanted to continue to work with the plants and in late 2012, she joined us, initially, for one month, which then turned into an extended treatment process with Ricardo and our team at Nihue Rao. After her first four weeks in Peru, Ricardo told her that she would have to diet for much longer in order to heal more completely. She decided to continue the process. She returned home and strictly maintained the *vegetalista* diet for four more months, after which she returned to Nihue Rao for an additional four weeks before closing what turned out to be a six-month-long healing diet.

During the first month, she stayed in a tambo in the forest, often in isolation. She was started on a diet with the master plant chiric sanango (*Brunfelsia grandiflora*), in tea form. Chiric sanango is a flowering shrub of the nightshade family with fragrant white and purple flowers. In the Shipibo tradition, the medicine of chiric sanango is believed to bring fortification to the joints and physical body (when dieted in traditional fashion). Maria reports that the first few weeks of her diet were primarily focused on working through a lingering heartbreak. She felt the plant medicine (her master plant and the ayahuasca) working on her heart, brain, and nervous system.

One night in the ceremony, Ricardo saw Maria in his visions. In his vision, he saw Maria in her tambo using diapers because of a vaginal discharge. The next day, he asked Cvita to go and check on her and see what was going on. Maria was shocked to hear about Ricardo's vision. She had developed a brown discharge and was privately using maxipads. She had not told anyone about this.

Around this time, Maria began to have strange dreams at night. In an extended diet, the plants often communicate to the dieter through dreams. She describes one dream in which "there was a prince in a dungeon, underneath this castle. This king was holding this prince and another child captive. Then I also had a dream of being in a car and my dad was there with me and I was in the dream giving him oral sex. We both felt really weird about it. Then he left and my sister walked up to the door of the car and she goes, 'What's wrong with you?' I said, 'What do you mean?' She goes, 'There's spots all over your face.' Then I looked in the rearview mirror and saw all these red dots all over my face."

Ricardo said that the dream was a sign that she was carrying a sickness from her past. In combination with the vaginal symptoms, the dream raised concern for repressed sexual abuse. In their ayahuasca visions, both Cvita and Ricardo had seen something related to such abuse. However, as far as the team was aware, Maria had no clear memory of sexual abuse. As Maria had not been the one to bring this up, no one on the team said anything about this to her directly. Ricardo remarked that there would be no benefit in putting such ideas into her head. She would need to see for herself.

Ricardo then decided to switch her diet plants to address his concerns, the discharge, and the apparent energetic illness in her uterus. He stopped the chiric sanango and started her on the master plant boa huasca (*Monstera spp*). Boa huasca is a reddish, woody vine known in the Shipibo tradition for its medicinal value in treating both male and female reproductive issues. Maria was prescribed one large glass of boa huasca tea in the morning and one in the afternoon. She was also instructed to use a bulb to apply the tea intravaginally, also on a daily basis. Ten days later, our assistant shaman Julian advised Ricardo to add ubos and abuta to her diet, to assist her further. Ubos (*Spondias mombin*) is a tropical fruit tree whose leaves are widely used in the Amazon to treat problems of the female reproductive tract.[1] Abuta (*Cissampelos pariera*) is another woody rain-forest vine referred to by some as the midwives' herb because of its longtime use in the treatment of all types of feminine ailments.[2]

In her visions, on more than one occasion, Maria began to see three horses that were all doing different things. The shamanic team determined that these three horses were her three plants. These three horses needed to be guided into order and balance so that their energies could work synergistically. In ceremony, the shamans guided these energies into harmony through song. Once things were in order, she went home to continue dieting these plants for four more months.

This four-month diet really changed things for her. She continued on a very simple *vegetalista* diet and minimized her social interactions outside of work. She reports that the diet "completely shifted my stress. My understanding of stress completely shifted. I had to live a completely limited life . . . I was [at first] on a diet where you eat sweet potatoes and rice and all that stuff [bland starchy foods, beans and lentils], and then I sent Cvita a message and was like, hey, I'm not losing weight. I don't know how good these foods are. Then she asked Ricardo. He's like you need to just do plantains and fish. So then I went straight to that, and after that my diet was way stronger [and I began to lose weight more consistently].

"My stress went down. I don't know how to explain it. This is the part where I explain it like the shift in the PTSD. I had had an amplified [stress response] . . . I was always on ten, but thought I was on one. When I was doing that medicine I realized that "one" is actually completely different than what you think it is. It totally got my body to relax in a completely different way.

"I started to experience states of anger and sadness less as rage and depression and more as 'oh there's some sadness.' I'm going to feel that. Oh, now it's gone. Instead of like I'm sad now so I'm depressed or I'm angry and now I'm going to kill you, emotional states completely shifted and I began to see a more balanced version of how I could experience emotional states. I realized so much of my trauma and my childhood, all that emotional abuse I had been dealing with and later to find out about sexual abuse . . . if anything triggered any kind of emotional state from my childhood I would enter a hyper-anxiety state. I didn't even realize it, because that had been normal. That had been the way people were angry in my home. That had been the way people were sad in my home. I'd never experienced any kind of 'normal' versions of those things."

After four months of the shamans' prescribed diet at home, she returned to Nihue Rao. Although she had had that disturbing dream about being in the car with her father, she still had not looked more deeply into the possibility of sexual abuse. At some point, when she returned, Cvita encouraged her to look more deeply into her childhood in order to find the roots of her PTSD symptoms.

During a psychedelic experience, gates are opened in the brain's sensory, emotional, and memory-processing centers. This opening may cause an individual to relive or regain access to previously suppressed memories and/or past emotional traumas. In the altered state, the individual then has the opportunity to process these experiences differently. Unrestrained, emotional memories interact with one another freely as in a dream, sometimes hybridizing into spontaneous insights and creative solutions.[3]

One night, Maria entered ceremony with the intention of going after the root of her emotional problems. Her first dose did not have much effect and then she decided to drink again. Before drinking her second dose, she made a commitment to the ayahuasca, "Hey, I'm willing to look at this." After the second dose, the effect came stronger and her visions opened up.

"That's when I saw all of the abuse. It took me to the various places [where the abuse had occurred]. I got to see the details. Then I met my little girl, who was living in this little box under the house . . . Then helping her clean out her house . . . Then, also, her showing me the rest of the abuse. That was such an important part of . . . She was like will you look at this? will you look at that?" Maria recalled. She had to see it all, opening the doors to her memories and her feelings.

At one point Ricardo diagnosed her with *susto*, loosely translated as "soul loss." *Susto* is a Latin-American concept in which a traumatic event causes such a fright that the soul, or part of the soul, is scared out of the body. This is more common in children who are particularly sensitive to such trauma. In one sense this detachment of a soul element could be described as a disconnection from one's inner child. This disconnection also manifests as a dissonance between one's conscious mind and the emotional body. Traumatic memories are suppressed from consciousness to protect the overwhelmed child. The inner child hides away. Perhaps the default mode network (DMN) is involved in such memory suppression. This suppression is an adaptive response, a form of protection; however, it blocks emotional processing. It closes the mind to the heart and body. It also creates blind spots in one's awareness.

In order to re-incorporate the detached element of her soul, she would need to regain the trust of the little girl "inside" of her. This little girl did not trust Maria. She did not trust that she would be kept safe. Ricardo let her know that her father's energy was still inside of her and that she would have to get this energy out in order to invite her soul back more completely.

"I went to ceremony to get rid of him. That's exactly what happened. In the visions, I went to different rooms, I blew mapacho, I took the house apart at the seams, but he just wouldn't leave."

In her visions, she negotiated with her father. It seemed that he was willing to leave in exchange for forgiveness, but there was still resistance. "When I said, 'Not only will I forgive you, but I'll get my mother to forgive you,' he left. Then when he left, we [Maria and the shamans] were able to take . . . I was able to take my little girl and put her back inside. When I did, she went inside me in a strange way and then I just asked God to help me put her in. Once she locked in, she went from child and then grew into a full adult," Maria recounts.

"In that moment I finally . . . It was like all of the missing pieces of myself were . . . I had never been whole. I hadn't been whole since . . . I had never experienced being that present in myself. I feel so present. Started to get memories from my childhood back. I had lots of blank spots in my memory, like holes. Years of my life I couldn't remember. All of a sudden I had access to all these childhood memories and felt whole again. It was like the rest of my brain, the rest of my being turned on, and I was there and present. It's been like that ever since.

"When I saw the abuse with my father that first night, all my trauma from my childhood made sense. It was like click, click, click. The bloody noses, night terrors, peeing the bed. All of a sudden every single issue I had as a child made sense. It clicked into place, because you're seeing the thing that caused all of that . . . All my checking out, living in a fantasy world, overeating, all these things. I would just see it and it was like click, click, click. It all made sense. In that moment. When I remember . . . When I had my first memory . . . When I put myself back together . . . I was finally whole. That part of me that needed to check out was not there. All of that was like shifted or gone.

"Then I had all this access to my memories and other things that I had felt like I had lost. That's been true. I have access to remembering my childhood now," she told me. This is a successful treatment of *susto*. The soul retrieval, which I theorize has something to do with the mind's conscious relationship with the emotional body, likely involves healing the relationship between the DMN and the limbic system.

Maria lost fifty pounds in that diet, and her back pain and knee pain improved. She also received extensive physical treatment by Maria Luisa, a traditional bonesetter who assists at Nihue Rao. Her mobility improved and most of all so did her symptoms of PTSD, which were rooted in unresolved sexual abuse. Two years later, she returned once more for five weeks. Then one year later in 2015, she returned for another three weeks.

At the time of her second visit, she was still having some lingering back pain, but overall things continued to improve. "The sciatica was gone. I was completely walking normal. I was able to exercise. I didn't have the inflammation. The depression is completely gone. I don't have those heightened states of anger. The skin rashes went away."

After the third visit in 2015 she realized, "I'm able to eat gluten again, which is crazy, because before if I ate gluten it would be, like, a hot mess. I was able to eat little amounts of bread. I was able to eat things that previously I had been allergic to. I still can eat them, but I just think that they are a little bit toxic. I still had a little bit of back pain and it's gone now. I don't have the back pain anymore now at all, really." (Food allergies are in part influenced by dysfunctional immune activity in the gut, which is in some cases connected to unresolved trauma in the emotional body.)

The last visit, as she reported, "was great, because that connected me to the anger and the emotional . . . all the emotional pieces I hadn't finished working through. Connecting to my anger. Letting go of anger and sadness and all those other things. It's been really helpful, because it's changed the way I experienced those feelings . . . now I can go into those feelings and let them go on a regular basis. It's healthier. It gave me more tools for staying healthy, for releasing things, moving forward, forgiveness, more tools on how to do that on a regular basis."

# CHAPTER 13

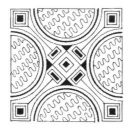

# Ayahuasca, TAPM, and Limbic Healing

No matter what humanity's future holds, we will never shed our heritage as neural organisms, mammals, primates. Because we are emotional beings, pain is inevitable and grief will come, because the world is neither equitable nor fair, the suffering will not be distributed evenly. A person who intuits the ways of the heart stands a better chance of living well. A society of those who do so holds a promise we can only guess at.

—Thomas Lewis MD, Fari Amini MD,
and Richard Lannon MD, *A General Theory of Love*

When Maria returned to the center after dieting at home for four months, she came to visit me in the office and gave me a book, *A General Theory of Love* by three members of the faculty at the University of California, San Francisco (UCSF) Department of Psychiatry. Maria handed me the book and said, "Here, read this, this is what you guys have done for me, you healed my limbic system."

In the book, the authors, Dr. Thomas Lewis, Dr. Fari Amini, and Dr. Richard Lannon, describe the process of limbic healing/emotional healing and its relevance in modern mental healthcare.[1] The limbic system is, once again, the emotional processing center of the brain, a central component of the emotional body. You might say that it is the place where the heart communicates with the mind. Through the limbic system, we connect to those memories associated with the sense of who we feel we are, defined by what attracts us and what repulses us, by our emotions, and our goals. The limbic system processes our emotional memories and gives rise to our dreams and sexuality. It is involved in our social and emotional connection to others and our attachment to loved ones. This processing system allows us, for example, to recognize the feelings expressed in the facial expressions of those around us, and other subtle cues that communicate mood and emotional state.

The more I learned about the limbic system in *A General Theory of Love*, the more I felt like I was reading about ayahuasca ceremony. Autobiographical emotional experiences, childhood memories, relationships, dreams, and sexuality . . . these were all the hot topics of traditional ceremony. As I gained experience at the center, I noticed that certain kinds of health problems responded more readily to the shamanic approach. As a medical doctor, I was looking for a physiologic link between these varied problems: disorders like PTSD, chronic cough, psychosomatic pain, and depression. *A General Theory of Love* provided me with the connection I was looking for. These problems are all connected to limbic system dysfunction, commonly caused by emotional trauma during childhood/adolescence and sometimes caused by emotional trauma later in life.

The limbic brain is described by some as the mammalian brain, as it is most developed in mammals. It is conceptualized as being seated on top of the ancient reptile brain, involved in more basic animal functions; and below the neo-cortical brain, associated with higher thinking and abstraction, most developed in humans. The limbic brain plays a major role in mammalian social relationships and, in particular, mammalian child rearing. In mammalian child rearing, whether in dogs, monkeys, cats, or humans, we see *attachment*, most obviously in the bond between mother and child. There can also be attachment to the father and to other early caregivers. These early attachments and relationships play crucial roles in our emotional development. These early relationships shape our future emotional and social lives.

We are, by nature, social creatures. Our emotions participate in an open loop system that includes those closest to us. During childhood, our emotions develop in response to and are regulated by our relationships with, first and foremost, our parents and/or caregivers. By tuning in to our caregivers, we develop our emotional selves. We learn to regulate our emotions through subconscious interaction with our parents and caregivers, through emotional cues. When there is a loud noise, for example, the baby becomes upset. The baby then looks directly at the parent for guidance. What should we do? Are we safe, are we unsafe? If the parent freaks out, the baby will freak out. If the baby sees the parent expressing calm, the baby will eventually settle accordingly. This emotional interplay, often subconscious, between parent and child, is constant. This connection is the basis for attachment and emotional stability. Through this social process, the limbic system is programmed, eventually influencing how we ourselves deal with stress, our future relationships, and our emotions.

It appears that our very identity, our ability to relate to ourselves, develops secondarily to our initial relationship with those closest to us. We relate to ourselves in the way in which we learned to relate to others. If there are problems in this process, if our early relationships are not healthy, then one might develop problems in relating to oneself, problems relating mind to feeling. If we are not accepted as children, we will have difficulty accepting ourselves. These problems result in dysfunctional emotional development, which often stays with us well beyond childhood. Such dysfunctional imprints, unless healed, often lead to lifelong emotional difficulties, ongoing problems with relationships, and difficulties coping with stress. Emotional trauma in childhood often leads to dysfunctional limbic development.

As we mature, we continue to interact emotionally and subconsciously with those around us. Further emotional trauma later in life, heavy trauma as in Russ's case in Vietnam, can also impact this emotional system, similarly imprinting us and disturbing our ability to relate to ourselves and to others.

The very social nature of our emotions continues throughout life. Instinctually, we constantly scan the emotional states of those around us, in part, for our own safety and well-being. In *A General Theory of Love,* the authors describe three concepts around the limbic interactions that occur between individuals in more intimate relationships. These interactions influence limbic development and functioning, whether it be between mother and child, romantic partners, or between therapist and patient. The first described interaction is *limbic resonance.* Two people can resonate with one another's limbic systems. By attuning emotionally to subconscious cues (through the eyes, face, tone of voice, etc.) that arise from the limbic system, two individuals can share deep emotional states. In this way they can tune in to each other's internal worlds. This is called limbic resonance.

Secondly, there is *limbic regulation,* which could also be referred to as mood contagion or emotional contagion. Once resonating, our limbic systems influence and regulate one another. In long-term relationships, limbic regulation affects the development and stability of our personality and mood. Limbic regulation occurs subconsciously, in childhood and beyond. Subconsciously, this regulation leaves imprints on our personalities and moods, which we then carry into our lives. Subconscious limbic imprints, for example, influence our choices in relationships. Someone who has been through an abusive childhood might end up seeking abusive relationships. For someone with that kind of limbic programming, it may actually be more emotionally painful to leave an abusive relationship than to stay in one. Dysfunctional subconscious limbic imprints lead to problems finding healthy relationships and make it difficult to center one's own emotions. These problems can drive individuals to seek mood-altering substances, as they look for a way to regulate how they feel. This external search often leads to substance abuse and addiction.

*Limbic revision* is the third concept advanced by *A General Theory of Love.* Limbic revision is the therapeutic alteration of personality through therapeutic limbic regulation. If successful, limbic revision leads to improvement in overall emotional heath, choices in relationships, and stress-coping mechanisms. Limbic revision is ultimately a subconscious process. In order to heal deep emotional wounds, we must engage the subconscious.

In psychotherapy, talking through issues alone may not lead to significant change. Deeper emotions and subconscious feelings must be accessed and addressed in order to stimulate limbic revision. In *A General Theory of Love*, the authors propose that in order for psychotherapy to be effective, the therapist must limbically resonate with the patient. This emotional contact allows for access to the subconscious. Over time, this can lead to limbic regulation and revision. In this process, it is most important that the therapist provide a loving emotional presence. Over a number of sessions, the patient will emotionally tune in to this loving reflection and resonate with this feeling. As issues are discussed, this reflection is maintained. In this way, the patient learns subconsciously to love themselves in light of their issues. This is limbic revision through love. In this manner, a loving psychotherapist can, over years, help to rewire the brain and undo dysfunctional developmental imprints.

Rather than seek psychotherapy, Maria decided to pursue traditional Amazonian treatment. Looking back, Maria felt that the combination of traditional ayahuasca ceremonies (guided by master shamans and their icaros) and master plant dieting led to limbic regulation and eventual limbic revision over a shorter time course. Shamanic healing with icaros is a form of limbic revision in which the patient's inner world is accessed through intuited cues and ayahuasca visions. In the dreamscape of the visions, the song works to revise what the shaman sees in order to restore harmony and inspire self-love. In Maria's case, further factors also contributed to her progress, including the extended retreat in a natural setting and daily access to a supportive community at the center.

It is worth noting that Maria was particularly dedicated to her healing. This makes all the difference. In all forms of medicine, the patient must do their part. She was very disciplined, committed to maintaining the *vegetalista* diet and continuing her master plants at home. When at home, she made sure to dedicate all of her extra time to herself, minimizing her social interactions, in order to process and integrate everything she was learning.

From the shaman's perspective, her deeper emotional healing required this prolonged purification and cleansing. Energies within her needed to be cleared, including energies/memories of her abusive father and energies stemming from her anger and grief. This emotional and energetic cleansing made room for profound healing and promoted a shift akin to limbic revision. Throughout this process, Maria entered a deeper intimacy with her own heart and soul.

Maria found this shamanic approach to be effective. Some of her prior healthcare providers had diagnosed her with a few seemingly incurable conditions: chronic depression, and chronic knee and back pain. She was told that, in all likelihood, these problems were related to her genetics and that she would need antidepressants and possibly pain medications for the rest of her life. Like most of us, Maria hoped for more. Ultimately she realized that what she really needed was deep emotional and spiritual healing.

Deep emotional problems, traditionally, are considered to be a manifestation of energetic and spiritual illness. Spiritual illness, soul sickness, manifests as limbic dysfunction, which some have also termed as neurolimbic dysfunction. Many of the people who benefit from psychedelic medicine and spiritual approaches are suffering from some form of neurolimbic dysfunction. This core dysfunction creates problems in the emotional body and is evident in depression, anxiety, PTSD, addiction, and many psychosomatic disorders.

The limbic system is the processing center of the emotional body. Mysteriously, this system responds to metaphysical limbic regulation, whether it be from a therapist's compassion, a shaman's song, or one's own self-love. We know that dysfunctional limbic development is commonly caused by a lack of love. We should not be surprised to learn that love is what can right the system again. Children need love, lots of love for their healthy development. Many people suffer as adults because they did not receive enough love in childhood. These individuals can, later in life, find ways to satisfy the needs of the inner child that lives within.

As we saw with Colleen and Maria, ayahuasca, the master plants, and shamanism together can help us to heal deep emotional trauma from our childhoods. Such spiritual healing techniques can help us to recover self-love and emotional health, thus guiding us to spiritual well-being. As I learned from Karl, this is the path to greater mystical access and, in his case, to understanding the nature of love.

# CHAPTER 14

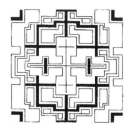

# What Is Love?

Spirit is memories, spirit is possibilities.

—Kogui elder, Sierra Nevada, Colombia

Sometime after Maria's visit, Karl, a seventy-five-year-old German man, visited the center. Karl is a very accomplished person with significant experience in spiritual practice and meditation. For decades, he has worked in Europe in the fields of personal growth and development, having served as coach and consultant to prominent individuals and businesses.

He came to the center with a couple of friends, one of whom had been with us previously. This friend had convinced him that we might be able to help him find what he was looking for. After years of exploration within his culture and beyond, including significant practice in Eastern spiritual traditions, Karl was still not sure he had "felt the spirit." He came to the Amazon to feel the spirit, as he heard this might be possible with ayahuasca.

As an experienced meditator and explorer, he was in general very comfortable with himself and his development. And . . . he was still curious, looking for something more; he wanted a tangible spiritual experience, an experience beyond his own intellect. He was well prepared and he entered the process humbly and with great patience.

We had screened him for medical and mental health issues prior to arrival and once again upon arrival to the center. I found him to be very mentally stable and in very good physical health, definitely above average for seventy-five years old. Like the others, Karl started his process with a plant vomitive and was similarly placed on a *vegetalista* diet. He also began a daily regimen with the extract of an additional master plant; in his case this extract was made from freshly ground piñon blanco leaves. Piñon blanco (*Jatropha curcas*) is a rain-forest shrub with large oily seeds currently being explored as a potential source of biodiesel. In the Shipibo tradition, the spirit of the master plant piñon blanco is believed to bring a very pure light to the heart and mind.

Karl arrived on a Sunday; once settled, his first ceremony was the following night. By 7:45 p.m., Karl and the others were seated on their mats in the maloka and the jungle night was in full swing. The ceremonial space at Nihue Rao is a large roundhouse approximately twelve meters in diameter. It has a hardwood floor and a tall, conical, thatched roof. However, there is no central post. Instead, its gifted designer, a local young man named Nilo, created a supportive spider web-like structure in the "rafters" that diffuses the weight of its sizeable roof. The maloka sits in a large clearing surrounded by a natural grove of nihue rao trees.

There were probably about twenty people in the maloka that night, including the *pasajeros*, Shipibo shamans, and "gringo" assistants. The guards were waiting for their cue to turn off the generator and everyone was quietly waiting.

That night, I was serving the ayahuasca. I was to decide how much to give to this "elderly" gentleman. I was cautious. As some Shipibos joke, "She is friend to no one." That is to say, ayahuasca should never be taken lightly.

At Nihue Rao, the ayahuasca is made exclusively from fresh ayahuasca vine and chacruna leaves. In most cases, this two-plant combination can be regarded as safe, although there are further considerations. As mentioned, due to the potential intensity of its physical and psychological effects, there is a risk of heart attack and/ or other cardiovascular events in vulnerable individuals (remember that Russ was screened by his cardiologist). As discussed in Chapter 7, mental state and history need to be assessed with care. Drinking ayahuasca requires significant psychological preparation and, furthermore, the capacity to thoughtfully reflect upon and integrate ceremonial experiences. Once again, one must also beware of potential allergic reactions and/or dangerous drug interactions. Remember that Russ was carefully weaned off of his Prozac and other medications before travelling to Peru.

By our standards, Karl was prepared. He was a good candidate without any significant medical or mental health history. Karl was not taking any medications. As the center is in a remote jungle location, almost no pharmaceutical medications are permitted while taking plant medicine, in order to avoid any unforeseen interactions. There are always exceptions, but these are addressed on a case-by-case basis.

I reviewed the possible "symptoms" of the ayahuasca with Karl, and then discussed the possibility of a visionary experience. I let him know that, traditionally, ayahuasca is drunk for healing, not necessarily to induce visions. For those who do experience "visions," the first level is often a sort of "psychedelic" experience, bright colors, geometric patterns, and fractals. Often, people report seeing the iconographic patterns brought to life in traditional Shipibo embroidery (called *kené* in Shipibo). These Shipibo designs are described as visual representations of healing plant energies. This first level of visions can progress in a variety of subtle directions, including spontaneous insights, memories, particular thoughts, and intuitions. As previously described, the world of ayahuasca visions can also involve more elaborate experiences, something like dreams.

Even in good candidates, though, an excessive dose can be more confusing than therapeutic. Furthermore, some people are simply more sensitive to ayahuasca's effects than others. I had reviewed this information with Karl and now it was time for him to try ayahuasca.

Ricardo the maestro was seated to my right, centrally on one side of the maloka, so as to direct the circle; alongside him were

What Is Love?          127

his artifacts and items. As he says, he sits there so he can see everyone, in his ayahuasca visions, in the dark. As I was sizing up Karl's dose, Ricardo was chatting in Shipibo with his colleagues, preparing himself for the ceremony. Ricardo glanced over as I poured Karl's ayahuasca. With some concern for his age, I dosed him initially on the lower side. Our goal was to find an ideal working dose, so that he could remain calm and conscious, so that he could *trabajar*, do his work.

Karl's first experience was mild. He described his first *mareación* as psychedelic, taking him to a state of consciousness that he had already experienced with LSD or other psychedelic substances. He saw colors and some geometric designs. He was hopeful but a bit disappointed, having travelled so far for just a familiar "hallucinogenic drug" experience. I prefer the term psychedelic over hallucinogenic, which simply means a substance that induces hallucinations. The term psychedelic is derived from the Greek *psyche*, meaning "soul," and *delos*, meaning "clear" or "manifest." Psychedelic could be said to mean something like soul-revealing.

Karl knew that ayahuasca contained the psychedelic biomolecule DMT and like many others had heard quite a bit about it. Many Westerners are very focused on the role of DMT in the ayahuasca effect. Some treat ayahuasca tea as simply a DMT delivery device, a primitive method for generating a "hallucinogenic" experience.

This contrasts with the Amazonian perspective. Ricardo and other *ayahuasqueros* are offended by this reductionist view, which frames them as drug peddlers. As Ricardo puts it, "We did not know one drug until the Westerners arrived." The *ayahuasquero* aims for something beyond a "drug" experience. The good *ayahuasquero* is pouring ayahuasca to facilitate deep healing through the master plants, allowing for the possibility of dialogue with the realm of spirit.

Despite his initial disappointment, Karl was patient and respectful. The *ayahuasquero* would call this a wise approach. Karl continued his diet and his daily process, hoping to get beyond a familiar psychedelic experience, hoping to truly enter the mystical world of the master plants.

His second ceremony offered him a bit more. He took a stronger dose and had a stronger experience, but still considered it a "hallucinogenic" experience, not what he would call a spiritual experience. Patience is eternal and Karl continued to wait for his chance to meet and greet the plant spirits celebrated and revered in Amazonian culture.

The process continued. Traditionally speaking, he was getting cleaner through the diet and the ceremonies. We reviewed his experiences in the morning group discussions and provided further guidance. He also processed some of his experiences through conversations with his friends and fellow participants. He was overall tolerating the ayahuasca well. As I remember it, it was during his third ceremony, after taking a second dose at around 10 p.m., that he began to experience what he had come to the Amazon for.

Ricardo often describes the second level of the experience as a form of personal review. In the end, ayahuasca is a mystical experience that does not require a logical sequence, but, for the sake of discussion, it is possible to describe a second level of the experience. Beyond the initial colors and fractals, ayahuasca may be inclined to show you your life, through visions, feelings, intuitions, thoughts, and memories. Ayahuasca may guide you to reflect upon and even relive certain life experiences, those that have impacted you most deeply and those that interfere with your progress. This might include everything since birth until now and, sometimes, experiences from before birth as well as future possibilities. This is where the bulk of the personal work occurs. This is where you work with ayahuasca to heal the story of your life, integrating your mind, body, heart, and soul. It is challenging, potentially difficult, and extremely rewarding.

In ceremonial healing at Nihue Rao and similar settings, the participant does not necessarily need to drink ayahuasca. At Nihue Rao and other centers, ayahuasca is offered multiple times per week. The *pasajero's* only obligation is to diet and to come to ceremony to receive the healing songs. Ayahuasca is offered for further healing and, as Ricardo puts it, "so that the *pasajeros* can see what the shamans are doing." By the end of the first week, Karl was on his fourth ceremony. He chose to drink in each of his ceremonies and he began, step-by-step, to find what he was looking for. In that fourth ceremony he had a direct experience with what he called spirit.

He connected with a spirit, presumably ayahuasca, who existed beyond his own intellect. To believe in her, he had to meet her. To get closer, he had to believe in her. This is the paradox of the mystical experience. To go deeper, we cannot simply wait for our minds to be convinced. We must let go of our doubt and believe from the heart. This is what opens the door. Karl achieved this and he rapidly grew comfortable with *la Madre* Ayahuasca. All of his prior mental and spiritual preparation resulted in a deeply profound dialogue.

At one point, he asked, "What is consciousness of consciousness?" Ayahuasca replied, "Love."

Lying in the dark on his mat, deep in the *mareación*, amidst the flowing icaros, he then responded, "What is love?"

Ayahuasca then guided him to a memory that existed beyond his conscious mind. When he was eight months old, Karl's mother passed away from an illness that may have been a complication of his birth. He did not remember her and, as a child, had been given only a vague explanation of her passing. The ayahuasca showed him something that he had never considered. At eight months old, when she was ill, he was often lying next to her in the hospital bed. The visions showed him that he was, in fact, there at the moment that she passed away.

In the visions, he re-experienced this moment, remembering it for the first time. Lying next to her, he sensed her passing and knew that she was gone. Like all babies entering the world, he was programmed and designed to receive support and nourishment, and now his mother was gone. He knew something was wrong and it seemed to be his fault. Like so many children who experience a trauma they cannot understand, when his mother passed, he blamed himself. He then realized that he had been carrying this guilt for nearly seventy-five years. This guilt was so deeply imprinted in his being that it had filtered the experience of his entire life.

It was then that ayahuasca answered his question more directly. She told him that love is the acceptance of all things as they are without reservation. The ayahuasca showed him that love was accepting his entire life unconditionally. In love, he did not need to take the death of his mother personally. He simply needed to accept and understand that her unexpected death was part of the circumstances of his early life. Within this acceptance, he could forgive himself for feeling otherwise, for closing his heart with guilt. The ayahuasca helped him to reach unconditional acceptance and heartfelt forgiveness, allowing him to love himself in a way that he previously could not. He had to relive this experience in order to feel its impact on his soul and in order to forgive. Forgiveness and acceptance allowed his heart to open further. The next step was to share this love with others.

There may be other ways to describe such an experience, given the altered state of consciousness and all of the other factors involved, but most simply put, ayahuasca guided him to love himself in a way that he had not previously imagined. She enabled him to experience love in a way that was previously inaccessible to him. It was then up to him to integrate this into his life.

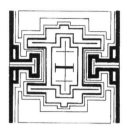

# CHAPTER 15

# Going Deeper with the Diet and Discovering My Song

*. . . if we do not remain humble and respectful before the spirits, those who would otherwise help us in the work of healing are likely to desert us.*

—Lewis Mehl-Madrona MD, *Coyote Medicine: Lessons from Native American Healing*

Over the first couple of years, I witnessed many inspiring healings at Nihue Rao. During that same time, I also observed as Ricardo guided several individuals through the one-year apprenticeship diet. This is the intensive training period required to become a *curandero*, a traditional healer, in his lineage.

By that point, I had completed three one-month learning diets with coca, but nothing long-term. I was balancing my time between the United States and Peru. Every three or four months, I travelled back home to work as a doctor, to raise more funds for Nihue Rao and pay my own bills. This back-and-forth schedule was not conducive to the training process, and at the very least was an excuse to delay. I was hesitant to train further, but things kept moving along.

Although I had not endured longer plant diets, I was gaining a lot of experience working with Ricardo and the other shamans. Ricardo continued to encourage me and, in light of my situation, he offered me a different kind of diet, one that I could maintain more easily while working back in the States. He called it the diet of divine light. Less restrictive than a master plant diet, one commits to no sex, no spicy foods, no dairy, no red meat, and no alcohol or drugs for six months or perhaps longer. Sugar and salt, vegetables, fish, and chicken are all allowed. This diet of light is a period of purification, a commitment to spiritual work, and an opportunity to strengthen one's connection to prayer. As with the plant diets, it was opened and closed in ayahuasca ceremony, and Ricardo offered some guidance along the way. I completed a six-month diet of light, partly in Peru and partly in the United States. This was, once again, a subtle experience, but nonetheless, a step forward.

By this point, Cvita had already committed to becoming a full-fledged *ayahuasquera*. She had achieved major breakthroughs in her training and was already doing shamanic work in ceremony, which included singing to Ricardo when he requested her help. Through her diets and under the guidance of our team of shamans, Cvita's powerful intuition and visions blossomed, informing our healing work.

Although I felt competent as a counselor, in contrast, my ayahuasca visions were diminishing in frequency and intensity. This is not uncommon. For many, the major visionary experiences calm over time. For the shaman, however, visionary access does help to guide the work. I was advised to try and figure out why I was blocked.

As in any small business, there were frustrations. I would sometimes squabble with Cvita over the way we were doing things. More often I would get into disagreements with Ricardo, complicated further by our cultural differences. We would always work it out, as we shared common goals, but I would sometimes hold a grudge, and this seemed to interfere with my ability to "see" in the ayahuasca. Anger, ego, pride, frustration, and impatience are all known to block the visions.

In the Shipibo tradition, shamanic vision can be improved through longer plant diets. Despite my occasional frustrations, I continued to feel the pull to explore shamanism further.

Given the intense schedule at Nihue Rao, by this time in 2013, I had been through many ayahuasca ceremonies, including a lot of very tough nights. Ayahuasca is a powerful medicine, and it is a very challenging one. Traditional Amazonian Plant Medicine can facilitate rapid gains, but those gains don't come easily. Many ceremony nights were tough on me personally, both physically and spiritually. Other nights were tough because of the work, the rigors of assisting others through very challenging experiences. At Nihue Rao, although we hoped for a calm ceremony, there were still the occasional bouts of loud screaming, flailing, and, unfortunately, the odd time that someone throws up on your feet (bare feet). Ayahuasca ceremonies get rough sometimes. The shamanic realms can illuminate us, and they can also expose us to considerable darkness: darkness from bad intentions, from the troubles of human society, from nature's destructive tendencies, and from mysterious sources.

Once particular night, when I was already rather exhausted, I had a particularly nasty experience with dark energy. Our work for that night was for the most part done; the *pasajeros* were resting. I was relaxing on my mat, coming down from a rather mild ayahuasca experience of my own, when suddenly, a thick, dark, hatred-filled sludge flooded into my visions, covering my body and spirit. This darkness weighed on my entire being like a heavy tar. Feelings of hatred poured over me and drained my will. I had no idea where this negativity was coming from but it flattened me. I sighed and rocked side to side.

I had not been sleeping enough as it was, and now buried in darkness, I was just too tired to do anything about it. It was just so dark and wretched. It was all too much; when would it stop. For the first time since starting work at Nihue Rao, I lay there in the dark and cried to myself. I was just trying to help people and learn about medicine and now I felt empty. As I had heard many *pasajeros* say, I said to myself, "This is it. I'm not going to do this anymore." All I could do was lie there and wait for it to pass.

Eventually—perhaps as much as an hour later—things shifted. The effects wore off, and I felt slightly better. I looked over and saw Ricardo relaxing. Thoughts of his life as an *ayahuasquero* came to my mind; I could hardly imagine what it would have been like to drink ayahuasca over and over again like he did. It just seemed so heavy, too heavy, and probably outside of my cultural jurisdiction. All I could think was, "What am I doing here?"

I told Ricardo about my difficult experience. True, I should have asked him for help earlier in the night, but by the time I realized what was happening, I was too far gone into the hopelessness. He smoked his mapacho and listened. I finished by declaring that although I was happy to translate, administer, counsel, and educate, I did not want to become an *ayahuasquero*. Becoming a doctor had already been hard enough—mentally, physically, emotionally, and spiritually.

Ricardo listened patiently. He then told me about the time during his training when he decided to quit. After a long and very difficult ceremony, filled with dark visions and negative feelings, he declared to himself and to the world that this would be the last time. No more ayahuasca. The next day, he told his master to remove everything, all of the master plant energies, the energies of his diets, and everything he had learned, so that he could go back to his "normal" life. In Ship-ibo shamanism, a master can help you to connect to the plant ener-gies and shamanic knowledge of your diets. It is also believed that, in a related fashion, a master can take that energy and knowledge away.

His master listened to his requests and then told Ricardo about the time(s) that he wanted to quit. Ultimately, he told Ricardo that he wouldn't remove the plant energies, the diets, or any of it. He told Ricardo to go and get some rest.

Ricardo then said to me, "It's fine, you don't have to become an *ayahuasquero* like me. I understand. You can be a doctor and live your life, *but* . . . learn the plants anyway. Maybe one day you will run into some people who are drinking ayahuasca. If you learn this, then you will be able to help them. Just think about it that way."

The morning after that ceremony, I ran into Martina, Cvita's sister-in-law, outside of the maloka. She is a lovely and intelligent woman with powerful eyes and a great big heart. After going through her own personal healing process at Nihue Rao, she joined the team and started working and training with us. I had first met her during one of my early visits to Iquitos, and she was aware of my journey. I told her about the difficult ceremony and about not going any further, not training to be an *ayahuasquero*. She looked at me and said, "Joe, this is your dream, this is definitely your path, this is your dream." I needed to hear that.

Over the years, Ricardo had helped me through a lot of personal healing, including emotional and spiritual trauma from medical school, trauma from some bad car accidents, and a slew of relationship issues. I had also seen him help many others. He was my teacher, my business partner, and also my friend. And he was right. I did want to learn more about this medicine.

I decided to enter the advanced training. I arranged things so that I could stay and work at Nihue Rao for an extended period, so that I could try a six-month diet.

## My Diet with Piñon Blanco

Ricardo recommended I diet the master plant piñon blanco. You'll recall that piñon blanco is said to bring a lot of light to the heart and mind. The spirits of its medicine are described as scientific doctors. Ricardo described them as being connected to profound knowledge in both the material and spiritual sciences. Sounds good, I thought.

I moved into a large tambo in the forest, initially built for a prior one-year dieter. It was a square, thatched-roof building, closed in on all sides with mosquito netting. When you rest inside, you can see the forest all around you, in every direction. And even with the netting, you can still feel the breeze. Over the months, the animals get used to you. The birds and monkeys and snakes wander by. The jungle night sings you to sleep. This tambo was a place where I could fully rest and reflect.

On the designated night, Ricardo opened my piñon blanco diet. I was still working hard at the center, in the ceremonies, and heading into town as needed. Through all of this, I adhered to the strict diet, no salt, no sugar, no oil, no dairy, no red meat, pork, or chicken (only certain kinds of grilled fish); no spicy foods, no sex, and no alcohol or drugs. I basically drank water and ate fish, plantains, rice, lentils, beans, and potatoes. I also ate apples and bananas, which although available were rather frowned upon among the Nihue Rao hardliners, including Ricardo (because of their sweetness). I continued to occasionally snack on these fruits for extra energy, with the excuse that I was working very hard, managing the center, often alone.

The first two weeks are the worst. Afterwards, your body starts getting used to the absence of salt. Eventually, once you get hungry enough, everything starts to taste good. Hunger is the best seasoning, as they say. I tell the *pasajeros*, as they start their diets, just pretend that you don't care about the food and eventually you get used to it. As Ricardo says, if you want to learn, if you are well decided, then dieting isn't so difficult. In the hopes of learning, you will go through the malnourishment and you will make the sacrifices. It had apparently worked for Ricardo and the other Shipibo shamans that I met. It was worth a try.

There are a few different ways to diet the master plant piñon blanco. Many people diet the leaves. Daily, the fresh leaves are ground and the resulting fresh extract is mixed with a bit of water and served in a small glass. One can also diet the resin. This is harder to come by as you need to extract it from the stem early in the morning. When dieting the resin, though, according to Ricardo's style, you don't need to drink it very often. Tobacco from half of a mapacho is soaked in water and then a small amount of fresh resin is mixed in. For the six-month diet, I only needed to drink the tobacco/resin mixture six times.

For me, the six months was again a rather subtle learning experience with the plants. The other long-term dieters spent most of their time in isolation, in the tambos. Dieters are generally advised not to talk with or touch anyone. They are to speak only minimally with the other dieters, the shamans, and sometimes the management. They are to avoid the distraction of social interaction.

This kind of isolation in the forest allows people to go deeper into their introspection. Over time, they become increasingly sensitive and this further opens them to receive information from the plants, which comes to them in their thoughts, dreams, and their occasional ayahuasca ceremonies.

Interestingly enough, in Ricardo's tradition, training to become an *ayahuasquero* does not actually involve drinking very much ayahuasca. After an initial cleansing process, for most of the year, the long-term dieters participate in just one or two ceremonies per month. The training happens through the internal relationship with the spirit of their master plant. As Ricardo says, they drink ayahuasca once in a while, so that they can see what they are learning.

Although I escaped this difficult isolation process, dieting while managing Nihue Rao had its own hardships. My opportunity was different. I could rest in my tambo here and there, but most of the time I needed to work. Beyond the day-to-day management, I would work in the ceremonies and drink ayahuasca approximately one to two times per week. Given all that and the fact that I was having few visions, it was really hard to tell if I was learning anything. I was busy and my mind was overactive. I was, however, clearly losing weight.

Cvita was concerned because she noticed that I was not receiving the kind of "downloads" that she and some of the other dieters were getting. She encouraged me to isolate myself more and encouraged me to be more about my relationship with the master plant. Ricardo also wanted me to focus more on my connection with the piñon blanco. After singing to me one night, he said he saw my piñon blanco off to one side, rather abandoned. On a separate night I also saw the plant. It was inside of me, but it was rather wilted, growing in a bucket.

In my mind, I regularly asked the spirit of the plant to try and understand my situation. Although I was busy and sometimes pre-occupied, I asked for some special consideration as I had by now given over my life to the promotion and practice of shamanic plant medicine. I was working as hard as I could. I listened to Cvita and Ricardo's advice, and I tried to focus more of my attention on my relationship with the spirit of piñon blanco.

Early on, I did notice something peculiar. A few weeks in, I told Ricardo I felt something around, I wasn't sure what.

He said, "A presence?"

"Yes," I replied. I felt another presence in my consciousness. I just had to quiet down and it was there, something was there. Although I was tired and physically a bit weaker, the longer I dieted, the cleaner I felt. Emotionally and spiritually I felt very good.

Although I continued to have only minimal visions, I did have some significant diet dreams while on this extended diet. One night I dreamt that I was talking to one of my medical colleagues, a doctor whom I had worked with in my *per diem* work. We had worked in an adjacent office for a couple of months, but I had never really gotten to know her. In the dream, I drove to an unknown building where I was to visit her. Dressed in a white lab coat, she greeted me as I entered the building.

During that diet, I had been feeling an ache in my heart and chest. This was related to my medical school trauma. Inside, I still felt like there was something wrong with me. I thought this was probably just some lingering sadness, but I wasn't sure. I hoped nothing physical was going on. I didn't share any of this with the doctor, but she already knew.

She whisked me away to an exam space and proceeded to put me through an extensive physical examination, which included opening my rib cage from the back to look at my heart, lungs, and chest cavity, all the way through to the other side. I stood next to her, also looking inside myself. She was pointing things out, here and there. As we explored, I could feel into what she was doing. Throughout the process, she supported me with love and kindness. Overall, everything appeared healthy and in my heart I knew I was well, I could feel it. I was relieved. Later I realized that this wasn't my old colleague, it was piñon blanco.

Toward the end of the diet, I had another memorable dream. Ricardo had once told me that when he finished one of his diets, he dreamt that he received some kind of fancy race car. Although he had never driven a car, in his dream he was somehow an expert with this vehicle. For him, it was the car of his diet, of his new medicine. With it, he could do things he had never done before. In the final few weeks of my piñon blanco diet, I had a similar dream of a big, lifted yellow and green hot rod. It looked like one of those high-performance drag-sters. I got in but I didn't know how to drive it. I tried, but I couldn't get the steering or brakes right, and I kept banging into things.

I told Ricardo about the dream and he said, "Oh, it's your diet, that's not good. It's not ready." So I extended my diet another ten days or so, hoping that I had not gone through the six-month process in vain. Then, during a ceremony the following week, unexpectedly, my visions opened up dramatically. That night, for the first time ever, I could see everything in the maloka as if it were lit up. I could see every person sitting or lying on their mat. I could see all of their faces. My closest friends appeared much larger than the others, two and three times their normal size. Over the course of the night, occasionally a green light would appear over one of them so as to draw my attention. I just looked around and tried to learn whatever I could.

## Becoming a Channel through Singing

One diets to learn the medicine of the plants and also to learn how to sing icaros. Learning to sing icaros is one of the mysteries of Shipibo traditional medicine. Hard to believe. I didn't believe it, but then it happened to me. I had heard stories from others, about how music came down pillars of light during ayahuasca ceremonies, or how spirits from the forest whispered songs to them in their tambos. For me, it was not so flashy, just a doodle in my head. I once read a book on drawing which recommended saving your doodles because they are a form of subconscious expression, unadulterated creativity. The melody of my first icaro came to me as a musical doodle, a little ditty in my head. When I was busy with an idle task, I would sometimes hear it in my head. Most of the time, I did not notice it, but it was in there.

Ricardo had some CDs of his own icaros that had been recorded during ceremony. Some of the apprentices worked to translate his Shipibo lyrics to Spanish, English, and other languages, (Ricardo would also teach us a few Shipibo words here and there in a lecture.) I would then use his phrases to piece together words to sing over the melody of my icaro. Eventually, I had enough of a structure set, with go-to phrases and a couple of melodic changes, to build a base from which to improvise. The idea was that, rather than sing something prepared, one needed to prepare a baseline structure, like jazz, that would allow you to engage the moment, to sing what you see. I tried to find time to practice in my tambo. I also practiced in the ceremony, very quietly, under Ricardo's icaros.

The words of the icaros all have a meaning and purpose. There are phrases, for example, about invoking the energies of the plants, opening the worlds of the medicine, and about cleaning the energy body. Through these chanted words, the shaman works to clean certain areas of the mind, body, heart, and soul. In the visions, problem energies can appear, for example, as a dark cloud or a skeleton-like spirit of the dead. Other times the shaman might see the *pasajero's* heart wrapped up in chains or notice a very burdensome energy weighing down on them. The shaman then cleans these specific energies, in part, by calling them out by name in their icaro. It is something like using song to interact with a dream.

On the last night of my process, Ricardo sang to me to close my diet and seal in the connection with piñon blanco. It was one of his last icaros of the night and things were quieting down. Afterwards, we all sat quietly for a bit and then he turned to me and said, "Okay, Joe, time to sing. Let's hear what you have learned."

That was my first initiation. He did not ask me to sing to anyone, just to sing my icaro to the maloka. The maloka was full of people who had come from all over the world to hear icaros from Amazonian masters. Like all the other first-timers, I was shy and embarrassed to sing. Everyone was silent. He was serious. I wasn't going to get out of this one.

I started my little song softly. I started with an invocation of the energies, "*Rama kano abanon.*" In Shipibo, this means something like now I am opening the energies. Then I sang the next line I had come up with in Spanish, "*ayahuasca medicina, limpia sana cuerpo*" (aya-huasca medicine, clean and heal the body). I repeated that line and then sang about the piñon blanco. At that time, I did not really have any visions, so I just sang about cleaning my body and strengthening my connection to piñon blanco.

After a few lines, I trailed off like a dying engine. Ricardo caught me falling and chimed in, "No, don't stop, it's good, it's good, keep going!" I would start up again and then try to stop, but he kept coaxing me on, "Keep going, keep going, it's coming along." He kept pushing me until I raised my volume and then, strangely, I hit some other level. I got into it. I started singing in a way that I had never sung before.

There was an energetic vibration to my voice and I started making mysterious tones. The ayahuasca guided me through the process, informing me through the feeling in my body. It guided me to become a channel for mystical energy, medicine energy. It started to feel good; the vibration pulsed through my body and I kept singing. After making a few more novel sounds, I settled down and stopped. That was the beginning. The plants had taught me something new.

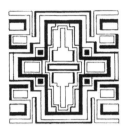

# CHAPTER 16

# Treating Psoriasis Spiritually

If you have a direct experience with spirit, it does change you—
it becomes part of your psyche, your nervous system. You recognize the unity of all things, you act directed by that, and it
modifies how you live.

—Chris Kilham, *The Ayahuasca Test Pilots Handbook*

. . . cytokines, messenger molecules produced by immune cells,
can bind to receptors on brain cells to cause changes in body
states, mood and behavior. That emotions induce changes in
immune activity is only the other side of the coin.

—Gabor Maté MD, *When the Body Says No:
The Cost of Hidden Stress*

As time went on, I continued to practice my singing, sometimes outside of ceremony and sometimes in ceremony. I
also continued trying to integrate what I was learning from
the plants with the scientific knowledge I was gaining through reading and in conversation with friends and colleagues. The plants were
teaching me how to sing to someone's energy body, which I knew was
linked to their emotional body.

Shamanic treatment often targets the emotional body, which, you'll recall, is comprised of the PNEI network that links the limbic brain, the autonomic nervous system (ANS), the endocrine system, and the immune system. Disturbances in the emotional body are often expressed through the autonomic nervous system and the immune system. As with Colleen's cough, such dysfunction can generate a number of inflammatory problems. Through related neurogenic inflammation, emotional disturbances can also exacerbate inflammatory skin problems, like eczema and psoriasis.

## Psoriasis and the Emotional Body

Sometime in the early years of Nihue Rao, a woman named Sharon came to us seeking help for her ongoing problem with psoriasis. Psoriasis is an autoimmune skin disease characterized by patches of abnormal skin. In autoimmune disease, a person's immune system attacks their own body. In the case of psoriasis, the immune system mistakenly attacks normal cells within the skin. The resultant inflammation causes uncomfortable psoriatic skin patches, which are typically red, itchy, and scaly.

From a Western medical perspective, psoriasis is considered an incurable disease that can, at best, be managed with medical treatments. There are different kinds of psoriasis, but plaque psoriasis is the most common form. Sharon had large patches of thickened plaque psoriasis on both of her legs. These lesions were very itchy and had troubled her for years.

Psoriasis is generally thought to be a genetic disease triggered by environmental factors. Symptoms often worsen during winter and with certain medications.[1,2] One clear sign that genetic factors predispose a person to psoriasis is that identical twins are three times more likely to both be affected than are non-identical twins. Psoriasis has also been associated with other problems in the PNEI network, including an increased risk of psoriatic arthritis (a related inflammatory problem of the joints), lymphomas (an immune system cancer), cardiovascular disease, Crohn's disease, and depression.[1,3] Infections and psychological stress are also known to contribute to the disease.[4,5]

In Sharon's case, there were apparent genetic factors. For a brief period, Sharon's father had had some psoriasis on his knee, but this went away on its own. Sharon's sister had also had a few similar spots on her skin when she was around nineteen, but this also resolved spontaneously.

Sharon herself was first diagnosed with psoriasis when she was also nineteen. She noticed a spot on the back of her leg, which later evolved into multiple spots. When these spots did not clear up, her mom advised her to consult with a well-respected dermatologist. This dermatologist diagnosed her with psoriasis and told her that, based on her experience, "You can't heal this. You'll always have it. What we can do is try to control the symptoms." Suffering quietly, Sharon followed the treatments, but did not expose her legs for many years.

Sharon's dermatologist prescribed tri-weekly treatments of UVB (ultraviolet B) phototherapy. Three times per week she would undergo what she described as a pretty dehumanizing process. As she told me, "You have to put a bag over your head and cover all the parts where you don't have psoriasis." Week in and week out, these regular clinic visits interfered with her work life, limiting her to freelance jobs.

Sharon's symptoms did improve with phototherapy. Her dermatologist also treated her with a number of different cortisone (steroid) creams. She did not feel well while using these high-dose creams and was concerned that they were thinning her skin. Although they were effective to some degree, once she stopped using the creams the psoriasis plaques would come right back. The underlying immune dysfunction in her skin smoldered on.

Her struggles with psoriasis drove her to become interested in "alternative" medicine. She consulted with a number of different healthcare practitioners. A naturopathic doctor linked her skin problem to her intestines, diagnosing her with "leaky gut syndrome." In leaky gut syndrome, abnormal bacterial growth in the intestines leads to increased inflammation in the blood and body. Sharon was advised to change her diet in order to improve her gut flora and was also guided to avoid pro-inflammatory foods.

Sharon studied books about nutritional healing and even became a vegan for approximately one year. She later tried to alter her diet according to Ayurvedic recommendations. Despite all of these dietary changes, she did not notice any significant improvement. Interestingly enough, her naturopathic doctor also treated her with topical Amazonian plant medicines, sangre de grado (*Croton lechleri*) and copaiba (*Copaifera officinalis*) oil. Unfortunately, these weren't helpful either.

She tried Chinese medicine for some time. Acupuncture reduced some of the inflammation, but she had difficulty taking the herbs consistently due to their foul taste. The TCM (Traditional Chinese Medicine) practitioner told her that according to her TCM diagnosis, her skin problem was related to anger held in her energy body (liver meridian).

At age 22, Sharon participated in a ten-day silent meditation retreat (Vipassana). After the retreat, miraculously, her skin symptoms completely resolved. In her case, spiritual practice proved to in fact be the most powerful medicine. Afterwards, though, she recalled, "I kind of went back to my life, and it came back." It was as if there were a tipping point in her system, related to her stress level, over which her skin symptoms would manifest. Despite a possible genetic predisposition, it did seem that there were ways to bring her body back below this symptomatic threshold. Her symptoms had also previously diminished on vacations in the tropics, when she spent a lot of time in the ocean, relaxing, and getting a lot of natural sun.

Sharon was well aware that she carried a lot of emotional trauma and that this was likely related to her skin problem. After a difficult childhood, she had suffered for years from anxiety and depression. Growing up, her father was angry and emotionally explosive. He himself had suffered sexual abuse as a child. Sharon described her mother as having been "unloving" and very anxious. There was not a lot of supportive communication in her family.

There was no real support for Sharon when, as a teenager, she had a confusing sexual encounter with her older dance instructor. When her parents found out about the experience, she was made to feel guilty. As she recalls, "We all tried going to therapy when my parents were splitting up and [her sister] went through her anorexia. I went and had the thing [sexual encounter] with my dance teacher, and everything was kind of exploding."

Sharon's psoriasis started during college, soon after her father's heart attack. At that time, she was in Washington, smoking a lot of marijuana. Her parents had been divorced for some time. Her father was living on his own, working as an actor in Georgia. Ironically, he was playing a character who suffers a heart attack on stage. One day in rehearsal, during a performance, he actually did have a heart attack. Initially, no one believed him.

Once at the hospital, he called on Sharon to help him. She travelled to Georgia to help him through his recovery. Later in her healing process in the Amazon, she realized that her father often called on her for her support and sometimes "dumped emotional stuff on her."[6]

Sharon later saw more therapists in college, but she did not have any luck finding someone she liked. She was seeking help for her family issues and wanted to address her sexual trauma. It wasn't just the sexual relationship with the dance teacher. She told me about a time she was sexually assaulted in college. "[There was] no alcohol or drugs, just the guy wasn't listening. We were out in the woods together. We were kind of dating at the time, but . . . we hadn't had sex before. I didn't want to, but he just kind of pushed it. That kind of thing where I'm not feeling really empowered to say no, which is kind of thematic of what happened in our family to some degree. It wasn't really an okay safe space to get angry or express angry emotions."

Sharon had been through a lot. She had been in a brutal car accident with her mom years ago and remained anxious from that. Although they both survived, during the terrifying ordeal she was convinced that her mother had died. Sharon also told me, "My abortion was really traumatic for me, the whole thing of the circumstances, you're kind of on your own, living your life. There wasn't a lot of support. I felt like I was talked into it." Sharon was holding a lot of grief inside.

She continued under the care of her dermatologist and as mentioned continued to explore alternatives. Then one day, from a friend, she heard about ayahuasca, a "weird thing you take, and then you puke your brains out all night." Her friend had told her that "it's like doing seven years of therapy in one night."

Before heading to Peru, Sharon had had the opportunity to participate in four ayahuasca ceremonies. She described the experiences as "pretty amazing. My first experience was really uplifting and beautiful. I actually saw myself flying on a bird leaving my hometown, heading south. I started having all these Amazonian visions.

"The next night [her second ceremony] I cried the entire night. I was very, very consumed by thinking about my cousin, who has cerebral palsy and had been really neglected. He was really emotionally abused his whole life, I would say. Never got proper care. My grandmother, my dad's mom, just kind of wanted . . . to . . . keep him down so that she had something to do in life that looked purposeful. That was a really hard night, but a huge explosion of emotions came [through]. The other [two ceremonies] were also [healing]."

During that first ceremony when she saw herself flying to the Amazon, she felt called to visit the jungle. She made arrangements to travel to Peru and visit Nihue Rao.

After her initial consultation with Ricardo and Cvita, she was started on diet of ayahuasca. Ayahuasca and chacruna are themselves master plants and can be dieted traditionally by taking small doses outside of the ceremony. When not in ceremony, she would take a spoonful of ayahuasca before bed, not enough to enter an altered state, but enough to influence her dreams.

Ricardo recognized that Sharon needed to connect more deeply with her heart and emotional being. He felt the ayahuasca diet would help her to do that. She was also started on some topical plant treatments for her skin. She cannot remember which plants, but recalls that they were not very effective.

After the first two weeks, she did not see any improvement in her skin. She was then switched to a diet of ajo sacha. Ajo sacha is sometimes used to clear energies associated with allergies, drugs, alcohol, and marijuana and, in general, to detoxify the body. Psoriasis is sometimes associated with atopic (hyperallergic) symptoms like allergic rhinitis and asthma. Sharon herself had some history of mild allergies, as did her father.

Her prior heavy marijuana use was particularly concerning to Ricardo. Sharon had smoked marijuana excessively for a number of years. In the Shipibo tradition, marijuana is considered a master plant (a spiritual teacher) and also a medicinal herb. However, like many other master plants, marijuana is known for having a dark side as well as a light/medicine side. (In Shipibo, the dark energies of the master plants are known as their *shitana*.) For this reason, the Shipibos believe that it is more responsible to consume marijuana within the context of a *vegetalista* diet. In this spiritually conscious manner, one is more likely to receive its medicine. If one uses marijuana casually and irresponsibly, without regard to its spiritual medicine, then one is more likely to accumulate the ill effects of its dark side (the *shitana*), which typically take the form of emotional congestion, lethargy, apathy, anxiety, and paranoia.

Used haphazardly, marijuana is believed to leave a sticky energy within the energy body. This energy clings to emotional traumas, holding them in, and slows emotional progress and development. In Sharon's case, to facilitate her progress, Ricardo made a plan to clean out this marijuana energy with ajo sacha, the diet, and ceremonial work.

During that first month, she had several significant experiences in ayahuasca ceremony. "What I started seeing was that my skin was just a cry for help. It was kind of like the voice that was saying, 'Please look at me. Please look deeply inside to really hear what's going on.'

"Then I started getting really clear that there was a lot of enmeshment, emotional enmeshment in my being. [Most of all], with my father. That I had taken on a lot of his emotions. That I had a lot of emotions stored in my body. It [became] very obvious that I had just been storing things. I hadn't fully been in touch with my emotions. I've always been a fairly emotional person, but a lot of it's because I [didn't express] a lot of it, when it was happening. A lot of stuff got stuffed and stored in there. I didn't necessarily know how to articulate or process each thing that had happened in my life. It just sat [in] there. A lot of my initial ceremonies were about feeling, really deeply, [and] having some really humongous emotional releases. Early on, Cvita had said, 'You have so much in your guts. There's so much there. I really see that you need to be here for probably one to three months.'

"Before going to the Amazon, I remember getting a colonic. I tried colonics for a while for the psoriasis. I remember the colon hydrotherapist saying, 'Your guts should be soft. Guts are soft, but yours are hard.' I didn't know that it was actually stored emotions in there.

"[During] a couple [of] very significant ceremonies, I did a lot of going to the bathroom and [purging] that way. [I did] a lot of body work on myself those nights, massaging my belly. The next morning, I had completely different intestines. It was really interesting. They were soft."

After one month, although she had experienced a lot of physical and emotional release, her psoriasis was not much better. She decided to extend her treatment. During a few of the ceremonies, the shamans had seen energetic problems in her uterus, caused by her sexual trauma. For the second month, she was switched from ajo sacha to the regimen Maria had been placed on for her uterus: boa huasca, abuta, and ubos. In addition to this preparation, she was placed on a diet of ojé (in the mornings, she would take a preparation made from its resin). Ojé, also used in the vomitive, is a master plant in its own right utilized for its physical and spiritual properties. Ojé is used as a gastrointestinal purgative and a spiritual cleanser. The ojé was added to further clear her body of marijuana *shitana* and toxic energetic congestion.

Over the first two months, in their icaros, Ricardo and the other shamans often worked on her childhood trauma. "I remember just going back in time. One night [in ayahuasca ceremony], I saw the dance teacher. I saw him and all the pain that he went through in his life. I had this huge sensation of [compassion for him], that I could forgive him because I saw that he was just really screwed up.

He had a really ugly past." The ayahuasca guided her to sympathize with him, allowing her to remotely *feel* into *his* emotional experience. After experiencing life in his shoes, she was able to open her heart to compassion and forgiveness. She released anger and resentment.

Over time she continued to progress. "I had this really big realization that the psoriasis wasn't mine. I inherited it ancestrally. Because I didn't have great boundaries. I'm kind of nice and kind of an easy target. I kind of let my dad step on me. Let other people step on me. I didn't fully respect myself. I wasn't fully in my own self. I wasn't even clear on who I was. I started claiming who I was, and that I was healthy. This whole path of getting healthy was so profound. This is true medicine. I am completely capable of healing and getting better because I'm looking at my deepest scars and . . . I have the power to heal myself." All along the way, she continued to discuss her progress with the shamans, members of the staff, and her fellow *pasajeros*.

As she healed emotionally, she started to notice improvements in her skin. At that time, Ricardo was assisted by another gifted Shipibo shaman, Marcelo Alvarez. Marcelo is an intelligent and open-minded *curandero*. Somewhere along the road (although he would not tell me where), he had learned that topical sulfur could be used to treat similar skin lesions. (I was surprised to later learn that sulfur-based treatments have been used for psoriasis in the Middle East for centuries.[7]) Jungle-style, Marcelo mixed powdered sulfur into Vicks VapoRub™ and gave the mix to Sharon to apply to her skin. The topical sulfur/Vicks mix helped a great deal.

"It was really the third month [after] we started using the sulfur and the Vicks. I started having this whole relationship with God that I hadn't experienced before. Replacing all this trauma and all the anxiety and the disease with God's light. I did a ton of visualizations and I learned that you absolutely have to let go, to let God in. That really helped my anxiety release because I just let down my guard. I was able to relax.

"Then, feeling connected to God, I felt like I had this ally that could come in with all that light and heal me. There was a lot happening, kind of spiritually and visually in my imagination as well. I visualized getting new calves. I saw a lot of angels. One time I heard the words, 'You have *Dios* (God, in Spanish). You have *Dios*.'"

Connecting to mystical energies gave Sharon hope. Her skin continued clearing, and then it regressed. "It kind of went back. I can't exactly remember what was happening at that time. I [started dieting more strictly] after that point. I [switched to] just fish and plantains for the third and last month. I really settled into being at the center. I think for the first couple months I was almost one foot in, one foot out. I hadn't planned on being in this intense environment for three whole months [on a] South American voyage . . . [Then], the third month, I said, You know what? I'm one hundred percent here. That was really helpful.

"Then I fully committed and things started clearing and clearing. [After three months, I closed my diets and left the center.] When I left, I still had some psoriasis. It wasn't until a few weeks later, maybe even a month later, that it just cleared. That kind of makes sense, because I feel like the psoriasis . . . it doesn't necessarily express itself when something stressful happens for me. It [comes from] the accumulated storage of it. It expresses itself later. There's some lag time.

"It made sense that my body was still processing all of this. [There was a lot of energetic cleaning to process from those ceremonies.] In addition to the Shipibo shamans, Cvita did a lot of healing [work] on me in the ceremonies, too. This was also very, very useful."

Sharon left the center to travel in South America and then two months later returned to volunteer and receive more treatment. During her time away, her skin had cleared for the first time in many years. True, she was in the warm tropics and enjoying herself, but she was not using any plant or medical treatments, not even the sulfur/Vicks mix. When she returned, she had only a tiny red spot on the front of one of her ankles.

During her second visit, she decided to ask for more help to heal the trauma associated with the car accident and her sister's anorexia. During this second visit, she gained a new perspective and learned about "how all of these things have affected my feelings about myself, my confidence level, what I've been able to do in the world. I think that the psoriasis set me back in a lot of ways. It kind of scarred my self-esteem. I spent so much time and energy working on that. It felt challenging to just be whoever I wanted to be because of this really uncomfortable, horrible thing that I was going through all the time."

During the second round of treatment, she struggled with anxiety symptoms. Ricardo recommended that she be treated more aggressively to clear out this anxious energy, which he felt was connected to marijuana. In addition to ceremonial work, she was prescribed multiple plant vomitives to cleanse this energy. It was the same plant vomitive that we used as our welcome cocktail, azucena with ojé, but with some added tobacco (mapacho) juice. Adding the tobacco juice to this mix can make this treatment very painful. Sharon made it through two of these very uncomfortable vomitives.

In this second round of treatment, she was also placed on a diet with three plants: ojé, ajo sacha, and piñon blanco. During this diet, she continued to have breakthroughs in ceremony. She learned how to observe her own mind and take a step back. From this perspective, she was able to recognize her thought patterns and "not get carried away." She learned ways in which she could better manage her doubt and anxiety.

Through Traditional Amazonian Plant Medicine, Sharon had worked to clean her energy body, her emotional body, her mind, her physical body, her guts, and her skin. Along the way, she gained a new compassion for the people who had hurt her in life. She learned to forgive and to connect to a larger spiritual consciousness. She also learned how to center and observe herself. She learned to recognize her thought patterns and the ways in which her emotions influence her physical health.

Feeling less burdened, she was then able to reconnect to her creativity, humor, and her interest in performance and teaching. She found meaning in her psoriasis. Towards the end of her second treatment, she told me, "I realize that I was given this as a gift [the psoriasis] to understand healing. To become a healer in the world."

"It was a very arduous process to go through. [Ayahuasca] was a challenging teacher. Ultimately, it was a gift because of all the things

I've learned . . . [I feel like I will] be able to help others now . . . I've done the work on myself. It starts from within. Then you go to your family. Then you go to your community. Then you go to the world at large. Become a light for others."

Sharon finished her process and went home, back to northern climates and temperatures. For eight months at home, with no further treatment, she was symptom free. The neurogenic inflammation that had previously smoldered under her skin, fueled by unresolved emotional trauma, had stopped.

She went back to her life and worked toward applying and integrating what she had learned. Then, slowly, after the eight months, as the stresses of life returned, her symptoms came back, however, less severe. The rash was less intense, not as itchy. She attributes the return of her symptoms to a return to the stresses of modern life in the United States. She is working on her career, her healing path, and has started a family. She is happier and continues to be hopeful. She knows that it is possible for her symptoms to improve and to even clear. Hopefully, as in Colleen's case, this will lead to continued physical improvement.

## Allostatic Load

You'll recall that dermatologists see psoriasis as a condition caused by a combination of genetic and environmental factors. There appears to be a threshold at which environmental factors push genetic factors into expressing the disease. Psychosocial stress, for example, is known to exacerbate psoriasis. Emotional trauma leads to lasting disturbances in the PNEI network, and this promotes the expression of diseases like psoriasis.[7-10] Because emotional healing can alleviate disturbances in the PNEI network, it can help to quell autoimmune diseases like psoriasis.

In Sharon's case, it seemed that the prolonged shamanic plant medicine dieting, the ceremonial work, and perhaps the tropical climate brought her system back down below the threshold at which her psoriatic tendencies become a problem. From the Shipibo perspective, this was achieved by clearing out accumulated pathological energies. As Ricardo says, people suffering from such emotional/spiritual problems need energetic cleaning. If they are not cleaned, they will get sick.

To paraphrase him, "They have all this stuff built up inside of them, but . . . they don't have a shaman, they don't have someone who can help them clean that out. Pharmaceutical medicine won't clean their energy body. Sure, when they're twenty they still feel pretty good, but by the time they turn thirty, they will start having problems, and by time they are forty, they're sick, they don't feel good anymore."

Does allopathic medicine recognize this shamanic concept of accumulated "energies"? I say, "Yes!" Scientific researchers refer to the burden of accumulated stress as allostatic load.[11] Allostasis refers to the way in which we respond to and adapt to stressful situations. Allostatic load refers to the buildup of such adaptations in our stress-response system. Some stressors, like low oxygen levels at high altitude, lead to adaptive responses in the body which help our survival. Other stressors, like modern warfare or self-esteem-eradicating advertising, lead to maladaptive stress responses in our bodies that in the long term don't help our survival. Maladaptive stress responses, if not corrected, accumulate inside of us and can damage our health.

In assessing allostatic load, researchers track levels of certain biomolecules produced by the stress-response system, such as cortisol levels, adrenaline levels, and certain inflammatory markers. These molecules are produced in response to stress and help to mediate stress. Once the stressor is properly addressed, once things settle, the production of stress-response molecules goes back down to "peacetime" levels.

However, if there is a repetitive stress, or too many different kinds of stress, or a stress that is so intense that the body cannot mediate it, the body remains in a chronically stressed state. Stress adaptations accumulate, many of them maladaptive, and allostatic load (stress related wear and tear) increases. If not somehow alleviated, the system becomes overburdened with these "accumulated energies," as we saw with Russ and Maria's PTSD.

PTSD sufferers are overburdened with increased allostatic load, exhibited by abnormal cortisol levels and abnormal stress reactivity.[12-14] Chronic Fatigue Syndrome (CFS) has also been correlated to increased allostatic load.[15] In CFS, the stress-response system is similarly overwhelmed. In Chapter 19, I will discuss the treatment of a woman suffering from migraine headaches. Migraines have also been connected to maladaptive stress responses.

Accumulated energies from emotional trauma (e.g., stress from childhood maltreatment, psychological trauma from combat) lead to increased allostatic load. Increased allostatic load represents overwhelmed and maladaptive functioning in the PNEI network, i.e., the emotional body.[14] High allostatic load and maladaptive stress responses leave us with less capacity to cope with stress, as we see in problems like PTSD, chronic fatigue syndrome, and migraine headaches. These are problems of the emotional body (the PNEI network), problems which Ricardo and his Shipibo colleagues would describe as spiritual illness.

# CHAPTER 17

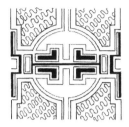

# Healing the Hurt at the Center of Addiction

Not all addictions are rooted in abuse or trauma, but I do believe they can all be traced to painful experience. A hurt is at the center of all addictive behaviors. It is present in the gambler, the Internet addict, the compulsive shopper and the workaholic. The wound may not be as deep and the ache not as excruciating, and it may even be entirely hidden—but it's there . . . the effects of early stress or adverse experiences directly shape both the psychology and the neurobiology of addiction in the brain.

It is impossible to understand addiction without asking what relief the addict finds, or hopes to find, in the drug or the addictive behavior.

—Gabor Maté MD, *In the Realm of Hungry Ghosts:*
*Close Encounters with Addiction*

D
r. Gabor Maté is a renowned speaker, author, physician, and addiction specialist. In the past few years, he has been speaking up about the positive outcomes he has seen in the treatment of addiction with ayahuasca and TAPM. In 2013, some of his

Canadian colleagues published the first North American study evaluating ayahuasca-based treatment for addiction.[1] This small pilot study demonstrated promising results and has paved the way for the larger Ayahuasca Treatment Outcome Project (ATOP), which is now being conducted in part at Takiwasi, a traditional healing center focused on addiction treatment in Tarapoto, Peru, under Dr. Jacques Mabit.

Latin-American-based research is now, in many respects, leading investigation into the healing potential of ayahuasca-based treatments.[2-6] Brazil, in particular, has become a focal point of this ayahuasca research. Researchers are currently investigating a number of topics, among them the therapeutic potential of ayahuasca in addiction.

In shamanic traditions, addiction is considered to be a spiritual illness, like PTSD, depression, or anxiety. Spiritual illness requires spiritually oriented treatment. Throughout this book, I have tried to demonstrate how what some see as spiritual illness can also be described in secular terms. When we speak about spiritual illness, we are describing dysfunction in the emotional body, measurable dysfunction. Modern research has clarified, for example, that addiction is associated with limbic system dysfunction within the PNEI network. Addiction appears to be a problem of the emotional body.[7-9] As we have seen with the treatment of other emotional body disorders, this, too, can benefit from deep emotional healing.

In his book *In the Realm of Hungry Ghosts*, Dr. Maté posits that addiction is a search for love (in response to a lack of love). He suggests that a lack of love during childhood emotional development often leads to long-term emotional instability, which then drives some individuals to seek "feel good" mood-altering substances as adults. In the case of cocaine addiction, researchers have demonstrated a strong relationship between early life stress and subsequent hypothalamic- pituitary-adrenal (HPA) axis dysregulation. (You'll recall that the HPA axis is a central component of the emotional body/PNEI stress-response system.[10]) As with psoriasis, addiction is likely the outcome of a combination of early life stress, genetic predispositions, and environmental factors.

In allopathic medicine, drug addiction is characterized as compulsive, out-of-control drug use, despite negative consequences. Instead of seeing it as a spiritual or emotional problem, modern science considers addiction to be a brain disease. In the United States, despite extensive research and massive expenditure, this "brain" disease continues to be a huge problem. The U.S. National Institute of Drug Abuse (NIDA) reports that the abuse of tobacco, alcohol, and illicit drugs costs the nation more than $700 billion annually (in costs related to crime, lost work productivity, and health care).[11] It is time to broaden our understanding of addiction and explore new treatment options. As we'll see in the following story, plant medicine offers promising pathways to healing.

# Mike

Sometime after Sharon's time at the center, in 2013, we were visited by Iron Mike, a big, strong, well-spoken Canadian in his mid-thirties. Mike is not a hippie or a New Ager, he's just a regular hard-working guy—an oil patch worker from Alberta, Canada who had a problem with cocaine. Unbeknownst to us, he had been doing cocaine all the way to the airport on his way to Peru.

As he told me, "Yeah, it progressed to the point where it was a quarter ounce (somewhere around 30 or 40 lines) a day, every day that I could get it. I don't know if I got some genetic ability to just consume unlimited drugs and live to be eighty or it was catching up to me, but the amounts I was doing and the frequency . . . I'm sure there would have been implications."

Mike first did cocaine in March of 2000. He described himself as a social drinker and mentioned that he had tried marijuana, LSD, mushrooms, and Ecstasy but denied having had problems with other substances.

"Yeah, cocaine was the excessive one. The first time I did it, I remember thinking very distinctly that I should never go near this again. It just had this effect on me. It was like the missing link. When it first hit my system, all of my insecurities, all of my inadequacies, everything that I felt was missing from my personality just came firing together at once . . . The very first time I consumed it, I remember thinking, 'Oh, wow, I'm going to get into trouble with this.'"

Over the next few months, his cocaine use progressed into a serious problem. Between 2000 and his visit to Nihue Rao in 2013, Mike had been in rehab four times, relapsing after every treatment. As he told me, "I would be sober for a period of time and then I would collapse. Everything I gained up to that point would go. Then when I got back to the bottom of the barrel, I would just check into another center or go back to another treatment place or go back to AA or whatever the case. As soon as I would do [cocaine], I would just instantly become fully involved in it again. I could pull it off for a couple weeks, little bit here and a little bit there, but it always ended up very quickly into 100 percent consumption."

In those years, his longest period of sobriety was just over two and a half years, from January 2008 until April of 2010. Throughout that period, Alcoholics Anonymous (AA) was a vital support. "That's where I had my most success in sobriety. [Consistently] . . . Not just stopping the use, but building some sort of a life through a connection to other sober people."

Mike was never treated with psychiatric medications, but in rehab, Mike recalls, "A psychiatrist told me I had borderline personality disorder and felt that it came from a lack of a father figure as a child. My dad wasn't around and when he was around he was really short-tempered and he just wasn't present as a father. From a very young age, I had temper problems, behavior issues, I had violence problems."

Mike's father was never physically violent with him, just angry. Although his father stopped drinking twenty-five years ago, he was an alcoholic during Mike's childhood. Mike's parents divorced when he was about eight years old, and although he always lived nearby, Mike's father was not a consistent presence.

"Yeah, I was just a kid without a dad. I didn't develop as somebody with a centered life. I didn't learn how to be a man at a young age. I didn't have that father presence. I just remember at a really young age I developed a temper."

Mike and his three sisters were raised by their busy, single mother. As he told me, "[My mom] had four kids to raise and . . . she worked a lot. She did the best she could. She was a really great mom." Mike's mother did not have alcohol problems.

I interviewed Mike in 2016, three years after his first experience with ayahuasca, about his visits to Nihue Rao in the Amazon. Mike had first heard about us from a friend back in Canada and decided to come down for a three-week visit. Like the other *pasajeros*, he entered the diet process in the usual fashion and was then started on the master plant ojé. Due to its strong detoxifying properties, ojé is often used in individuals with alcohol and drug problems. Once prepared, Mike entered ceremony. To put it lightly, his first couple of ceremonies were challenging.

"During the first night, like the fool I am, I went up to the well [to drink ayahuasca] twice and ended up in that other [*pasajero's*] bed. I completely ruined their night. I didn't know the bed from the floor. I had no experience with this stuff and definitely had no business helping myself to two [doses].

"I was completely disoriented. Being the addict I was, when I went up there, I remember you asking me, 'Are you feeling the effects?' and I was like, 'Oh, no, not really.' I was [feeling the effects], right, but if I say I am, they're not going to give me more, so I just completely BS'd my way into another round and I think that was part of the payback for being greedy.

"Yeah, I was detoxing still. I remember I had a drink on the plane on the way down there and was buying painkillers at the airport in Lima. They don't care there, they'll sell you anything. Whatever they got on the rack is up for grabs. Once me and the pharmacist established what I was trying to get he just handed it right over . . . the first night [of ceremony], I was still coming off of a really rough thing. I just got greedy and got leveled for it.

"I couldn't even get off the floor. I couldn't see, I couldn't find my bed. I just remember lying there and thinking, 'Man, am I ever helpless right now?' This is bad. I knew I had overdone it. I had this feeling of that's what you get.

"The next ceremony was much different. That was the night I was lying there and I heard this voice and I thought you [had] just snuck up on me, and I was just sitting there looking around and nobody was there. That's when I realized something is trying to guide me here. I was trying to be rational. I had this moment where I was like, 'Okay, there is nobody around you, you need to calm down a minute here and just go with this and not try to figure it out.'

"If I could [have] just put some rational thought to this, I thought it would make sense. That wasn't the case. There was no putting any rational thought to it. I remember I had this feeling of, 'Man, you're in the jungle now.' This thing is coming alive. I had this moment of clarity where I could hear all the noises in the Amazon and I was like, 'Oh my goodness, I'm in South America, I'm in the middle of the Amazon jungle and this voice just kicked in. I'm going to be here for three weeks, I better get comfortable here and quickly.'

"The first ceremony, I was just a write-off, but when that voice and that sort of guidance came in, right away it gave me an offer. It was like, you have a choice here, if you're down here to change, you're going to have to experience some painful things. Or you can go on living the way you're living. I had this option at that moment to make a decision, and I decided to proceed forward.

"[So] what happened that night was that a line-up of ex-girlfriends showed up. My ex-wife, my ex-girlfriend, I was lying there and, one by one, they appeared in front of me crystal clear as if they were standing there. They explained to me what my actions had done to them, how it had hurt them, how it had affected them, how it affected their lives, and how it had made them feel about themselves. It was four or five of them in a row. It was not easy, man. That was a rough road."

Mike did not feel that he was guided through these experiences to make him feel guilty, "but in order to understand things I needed to have the severity and the seriousness of it put to me, and the best way to do that, in that moment, was through a visual interpretation of it. That's what I got. I wouldn't have known any different if they were standing right there yelling at me. It was that clear. I was looking and they were physically there, standing there and letting me have it.

Nobody took it easy on me that night. That was a tough night in the jungle.

"At the end of that, I remember thinking, 'How am I going to get through three weeks of this? This is ridiculous. Nobody told me about this.' Then there was a break [a night off, after the first two ceremonies]. Everything that I had to feel from that [second] night just stuck with me. It didn't leave. There was no reprieve granted that night and I think that was intentional. You need to sit with this. You're not just going to say, 'Here's where you went wrong and now you feel better about yourself.' That night and the next day and into the following day, right up until [the next ceremony] night, my heart was just heavy. It was just the weight of the world on me. Not in the sense of self-pity or sympathy, it was just I was feeling the pain I had inflicted on others. I was really connected to what my actions had done to other people.

"It was tough. I woke up the next morning and I was like, 'I hate myself.' I don't even know if I slept. I think I just lay there all night feeling sorry for myself. This is wrong, man. I haven't been through anything like that.

"It was kind of put to me from that point on. In between the bathroom breaks and all the crying and sweating, and the stuff that goes on when you're cleaning out, I learned a lot about why I was unhappy. Why I was self-destructive, why I was counterproductive to my own future.

"I learned that it was because of my selfish behavior . . . When I hurt somebody that I loved out of selfishness, I would turn that into self-anger . . . to beating myself up and saying I'm a bad person, because I have a conscience. If I didn't have a conscience, like your average sociopath, it wouldn't have been a big deal. I would have just moved on to the next one. I truly cared. I was completely unable to stop the cycle that I had created for myself. Lying, cheating, deceiving, and then self-hatred and self-loathing. That would manifest into drugs and alcohol and lot of other behavior and all the other things that would come with it. Once I would see the effect I was having on people and my conscience would get to me, I would just medicate and self-destruct and it would just feed itself. When I was behaving like that, I was hurting the people I cared about even more. It would just constantly be this wheel that was fed with negativity.

"One of the very early fundamentals I learned [from] working with this plant was that 'if I'm going to hurt other people, I'm going to hate myself. If I'm going to hate myself, then I'm going to self-destruct and I'm never going to be happy.' It starts with, in my case, the way I'm treating the people that I care about. Even the people that I don't care about."

After two days in the jungle with a heavy heart, reflecting deeply on his realizations, Mike entered his third ceremony.

"I dragged my sorry ass in there feeling . . . like, 'Oh man, what's coming? Not another one of these . . . ' The heaviness that I felt in my heart, that voice came back and was like, 'You're going to remove this. Now that you understand what you're doing. Now it's time to start caring about yourself.' That next ceremony, after the Wednesday break, was when the guilt, the shame, the remorse, all that stuff started to come out of me. When I was able to really get the weight lifted out of my heart.

"The real crazy one would've been the fifth or sixth ceremony. They came and got the guy beside me and brought him up [to the shamans], then Ricardo said something and they brought the guy back." The helper had brought Mike's neighbor, but in that particular moment, Ricardo changed his mind and decided that he specifically wanted to sing to Mike. Deep in his ayahuasca effect and a bit confused over the shuffle, Mike allowed the helper to guide him over to Ricardo.

Mike continued:

"[I was brought up in front of Ricardo for the icaro and] there was a crazy moment where [Ricardo] kind of sat up and leaned in on me and started making these really weird noises. I felt like my chest had opened up and something was being pulled right out of it. The weight of this darkness, it was just like he sucked it right out of my chest. I couldn't feel my legs. This went on for ten minutes. When I went back to my [mat], I could barely walk. I was like, 'Holy [smokes], is that an exorcism? What just happened there?' I felt like he had just taken that negativity, [in] that moment [he] just saw the opportunity to take something out of me and clean me. That was the real changing moment.

"I had been feeling good up to that point, because it was five or six ceremonies in, but after that night, was the point that I knew that my path had forevermore altered. I felt like from this point on you have a choice."

The power to choose, improved personal agency, improves personal mastery and, with it, spiritual well-being and emotional body function.

"Up to that moment in my life, I just didn't feel I had any choice over how I was behaving. I was completely unable to stop the bad behavior. That night I remember when I got back to the mat and [then] back to my hut, I remember thinking, 'From this moment on, you can choose if you want to be that person, or you can choose if you want to be a better person.' It was just so clear, for the first time in my life I now had the option. Does that mean everything is going to be perfect? No. It's just that I didn't have a choice before. I could never stop the behavior."

I mentioned to Mike that I had come across a quote that said, "Once a person discovers a mystical or archetypal experience in his memory banks, he never again can view himself as worthless—which might well prove to be the most potent contribution of entheogens [psychedelics] in the treatment of addictions."[12] I wanted to hear his perspective on this idea, that a major mystical experience can help an addict transcend the feeling of worthlessness, that on the other side of worthlessness is choice.

Mike responded, "What's going on with everything since my first visit down there is that I have the option if I want to keep suffering. I have the option if I want to get better. I firmly believe that I have the option . . . I really believe that sort of set off that night. I really believe that was the big catalyst."

Mike finished the three-week experience feeling "amazing." In his own words, "Things had been so bad for so long that part of my final experience in those final ceremonies was just to learn how to feel good and enjoy feeling good and enjoy taking some positive lessons . . . The punishment stopped."

Mike had to go through his own forgiveness and acceptance process in order to move forward. "That was one of the keys to this thing. I had to understand it. It wasn't because I was a bad person. It was the situation. It was a sickness. To come to accept all those things."

Unfortunately, once home, he learned that he had come down with malaria.

"I was halfway to getting home, on the plane and I was like, 'What is going on? Something is not right.' I thought it was jet lag but after about the third day I was like, 'This is not normal.' [Mike went to see his doctor and was diagnosed with malaria.] But the thing was, when they treated me for it, the next day everything just returned. Once the malaria was gone, how good I felt, that all returned, it was just a sickness. It came and went. It didn't affect me spiritually."

Six months after his first stay, Mike sent me an email saying, "It's now nearing the end of December, and six months later. So what has become of the man who lost his soul and begged for mercy from the plants of the amazon? My life, and the very existence I've ever known, has been completely transformed. I have experienced things in the last six months that I would never have believed possible. I live a caliber of life that people would die for. I am clean, sober, healthy, and most of all Joe. I love myself."

Not too long after that email, Mike decided to go back to work in the oil patch. A few months later, approximately nine months after his stay at Nihue Rao, he started using again.

During the 2016 interview, Mike recalled, "Yeah. I had forgotten the fundamentals that I learned as far as what was important. Because I had never felt that good in my life, I got complacent. It started out with going to the pub with friends and drinking and thinking, 'Well I'm cured, I've got this thing beat.' It was a situational thing and I can drink and behave like this again. Sure enough it didn't take long from when I started drinking again until the cocaine came back. Then again it just fell apart very quickly. It just collapsed again."

Yes, Mike relapsed, but things never got as bad as they had in the past. He was able to overcome his self-hatred. He still had the power to choose, and he realized he needed more help. Mike's mother advised him to return to Nihue Rao. He returned in April of 2014 for two more weeks. Ricardo started him on ajo sacha for this two-week diet, another plant used in cleansing the body of addictive substances. This two-week trip quickly got him back on track.

I asked Mike how he felt after his second experience. He replied, "Oh, yeah. I was doing incredible. I think what made that trip magical was the group of people that I met down there. All those guys and we just formed a really tight friendship very quickly. We had a really great time together. . . . It really restored me, being back there that time.

"Again, things were going so well. [When I got back to Canada] I went back to the oil and gas industry, which in the divisions I was working was very high pressure. [You're] working with people with tempers, there is a lot of backstabbing, there is a lot of fighting. You can't really be a pacifist . . . You have to just be a bull to get things accomplished and survive . . . I kind of fell back into that role again."

After another seven or eight months of working in this environment, Mike started using cocaine again.

"After I left Peru, I never did anything to maintain sobriety. I just rode the wave of [good feelings] without reconnecting to something. For the second time, I just thought, 'Man, I'm fixed. I just had a little bit of a dustup there, but I'm back on and it's all good.' Again, there was no maintenance of spiritual condition. I just kind of came back and went back to living the life, with the oil fields, and the trucks, and the money, and all that stuff."

After this relapse, Mike returned to the center for one more week and then followed up by taking an opportunity to participate in ayahuasca ceremony in Portugal.

"We worked really well in Portugal. One of the things that I hadn't dealt with was the loss of my marriage. I had never really forgiven myself. I had never come to terms with it. I hadn't allowed myself to go through the feelings of it. How much that really meant to me, how much that really affected me for that to have happened.

"That happened six years ago. [Mike was married in July of 2009 and got divorced in May of 2010.] The weight of my decisions that cost me that opportunity, that cost me that partnership, I never really allowed myself to understand how deeply I felt about it. [My wife] wasn't into drugs or anything like that. She supported me in sobriety and supported me going to AA and being around sober people, but when the relapses happened, when I wasn't ready to stop it, she gave me more than enough opportunity to put the brakes on it and to get better and reach out for help. When that wasn't happening, she just couldn't be around it."

Mike worked through forgiving himself and is now most focused on applying what he's learned from his experiences with master plants.

"In spite of the treatment I received with the plants and the different ceremonies I went to, when I got home, I didn't put any action into continuing the connection. Although I had been able to bounce back from setbacks, what has held me up was that I didn't put the effort into staying connected to something other than to just go back to my complete old lifestyle and expect everything to change."

After Portugal, Mike started using again for a period of time over the winter but was able to pull out of it on his own, with the help of his community. When we last spoke, he was back on track again.

"When I was telling you today about what's going on [over] the last few weeks, me being able to be in the situation I'm in right now and doing as well as I'm doing in the brief period of time, that I swung back, this would not have happened in my history . . . I wouldn't have been able to stop. It would have had to get to the point where [I needed an intervention,] a treatment center . . . [or] going back to Peru.

"What I'm finding now that I'm in AA and working with people that are spiritual people and people that are clean and sober, when I'm living around people that are living in the solution that I want to be a part of, I'm finding the solution is becoming a part of my everyday life. Instead of being back in the oil fields, instead of being back around people that are drinking, back around people that are around drug dealers, back around all that, just expecting to maintain this great thing . . . That's the big thing. That's the big deal. It's a boost. It's a day-to-day thing, it's real life. To stay connected."

At first glance, it might seem that ayahuasca and the TAPM treatment failed to heal Mike. But that's not what Mike took from the experience.

After maintaining his sobriety for some time, Mike spoke with a therapist who has seen others go through plant medicine experiences. Mike told me that this therapist said something to him like this:

"You can go down to the Amazon and do a night banger through the jungle and have a great time and be safe, but if you don't understand the messages that are being given and find a way to apply them in your life, all you are doing is going on a rodeo tour. When you come back, you're left with all these answers and you're not connected to anything. There's a whole other side to this that isn't just about drinking the medicine and expecting to be fixed.

"We go down there because we are in such bad shape and we come back having never felt so great about things. We forget that there is work needed to maintain this stuff. You're not going to feel great forever, but there is a way to consistently be dialed in, and it involves some work outside of going to Peru once a year. You can't just expect it to be fixed."

Mike is now part of a healthy community, working part-time as a firefighter, and interested in getting back into radio broadcasting. In his new community, he attends AA meetings regularly.

"This is the first time since I've visited Peru, since before I went to Peru, that I have the understanding that I need to be connected to something that is going to keep me sober. I'm not going to stay sober based on the fear of my last bad experience. Fear is not going to keep me sober. Fear of relapsing isn't going to keep me from relapsing. One thing to keep me from relapsing is putting in some work. Without what happened in Peru and the experiences I have had . . . well, [I can say that this plant has] taught me to how to fight instead of just roll over and die and give up. There is always another option, a lot of hope.

"Before I didn't have the choice. I didn't have the choice when I relapsed . . . Now I have the option. I know what needs to be done,

I know how I can feel about myself if I put the work in and I know where to get help if I want it. I know that I'm worth fighting for. Before, [that] wasn't a part of my psyche, it wasn't a part of my thought process."

Mike and I are now friends, and I hope to be on his radio show one day. He is still going to AA meetings and he is still sober.

# Mystical Healing

Although Mike's path to sobriety was long and complicated (involving multiple plant diets and ongoing social support), he is quite clear that the ayahuasca ceremonies opened the door to his transformation. His mystical ceremonial experiences were crucial to uncovering and healing the deep emotional wounds that were preventing his success. We are now discovering more and more about how such mystical experiences shift perspective and help someone overcome the feelings of worthlessness that underlie self-destructive behavior.

Dr. Roland Griffith's research group at Johns Hopkins Medical School (Dept. of Psychiatry) is currently investigating the role of mystical experiences in healing.[13-15] They are using psilocybin-induced states of consciousness as a model for the mystical experience, exploring the way mystical states affect healthcare outcomes.

In their research, they use a secular scale, The Mystical Experience Questionnaire, to try and determine how "mystical" a particular psilocybin experience was. This scale is a subjective questionnaire that explores the degree to which a study participant, for example, had the experience of feeling eternity or infinity, or the experience of fusion with a larger whole, or the feeling that they had gained insightful knowledge at an intuitive level, etc. Using their Mystical Scale and other research instruments, researchers have found that those psilocybin experiences rated as more mystical were also found to be more personally meaningful and spiritually significant, and that personally meaningful and spiritually significant experiences promote more lasting change.

This aligned with prior observations that I had read: "Naturally occurring instances of dramatic, positive behavioral change are sometimes associated with spontaneously occurring transformative psychological experiences, frequently of a mystical-type variety and with prior psychedelic research demonstrating that mystical-type experiences, transcendent or peak experiences, played a key role in positive therapeutic outcomes (including early research investigating the treatment of drug and alcohol dependence and, more recently, the treatment of anxiety associated with advanced cancer)."[14]

The Johns Hopkins group applied these concepts to a further study investigating a psilocybin-based treatment for tobacco addiction.[15] In an attempt to get them to quit smoking, fifteen people were put through a treatment program that included up to three clinically observed psilocybin experiences. After the treatment program, twelve of the fifteen study participants quit smoking. Six months later, those twelve were still not smoking. The participants who quit smoking reported stronger mystical experiences with psilocybin and rated these experiences as more personally meaningful and spiritually significant as compared to those who did not quit. The investigators summarized, "These results suggest a mediating role of a mystical experience in psychedelic-facilitated addiction treatment."

Why the science "talk" again? Well, apparently, tobacco addiction, a "brain" disease, regarded commonly as a physical addiction, can be "mediated" by a mystical experience. Mike's cocaine addiction was similarly affected by his mystical experiences with ayahuasca. Perhaps it is time to expand our understanding of addiction. "Brain disease" doesn't seem to quite cover it.[16]

Profound, mystical experiences of self-love can apparently reprogram the mind-body in a meaningful and lasting manner. Mike's experiences in ayahuasca ceremony helped him to overcome much of his deep emotional suffering, so that his story could be retold and his brain could be "rewired." This transition was further facilitated by shamanic healing, master plant diets, subsequent integration, and social support.

Feeling is what affects the emotional body. Sometimes the master plants and the energy of an ayahuasca ceremony can make you feel something so strongly that it can change your life. Such experiences can even impact something as physically intense as cocaine addiction. Ayahuasca helped Mike cross into the mystery to find and fully feel self-love, forgiveness, compassion, and gratitude. These faculties of the soul then promoted healing in his emotional body, which then translated into changes in his mind-body.

Afterwards, clearly, there was more work to do. Traditional medicine all over the world acknowledges this. After traditional healing, if you don't change your life, nothing will change, not for long. You have to do your part to maintain a shift in the emotional body. If you don't, your mystical Amazonian experiences will fade into that memorable "rodeo tour," that one time, in the jungle.

# CHAPTER 18

# Plant Protection and Finding a New Song

True realism consists in revealing the surprising things which habit keeps covered and prevents us from seeing.

—Jean Cocteau

Sometime after Mike's first visit, I entered my next learning diet. I had planned to be at the center for several months, in part, so that I could move forward with my next three-month diet. Ricardo suggested that I diet bobinsana (*Calliandra angustifolia*), a shrubby tree that produces beautiful, pink and reddish powder-puff-like flowers. Outside of shamanism, bobinsana is used as an herbal medicine for a variety of ailments, including joint pain and rheumatism.

Under Ricardo's direction, we had planted a number of bobinsana trees in a ring around the maloka at Nihue Rao. At the time of my diet, they had matured and were flowering regularly. They were planted as a form of spiritual protection, as this plant's spirit is believed to be protective against malevolent energies. Ricardo suggested that I diet this master plant to learn from the spirit of its medicine and, in part, for my own protection in our shamanic work. There are risks associated with opening up shamanic realms in ayahuasca ceremony. Ricardo told me that bobinsana could make me invisible to dark energies and to those who might try to harm me spiritually. In addition to this protection, I hoped to progress in my shamanic practice and with my icaros.

As before, Ricardo opened my diet in ceremony and I continued my normal work at the center. I maintained the *vegetalista* diet and, once a day, drank a fresh extract made from the leaves of the bobinsanas growing around the maloka. This diet, further into my apprenticeship, was different from the piñon blanco diet. During my bobinsana diet, I had more frequent visionary experiences in ceremony and was occasionally receiving information and ideas. Things can get pretty strange at an ayahuasca healing center, and on this diet, things seemed to get even stranger. During one ceremony, a *pasajero*, an older gentleman from California, "saw" me disappear right in front of him. I had just walked him back to his mat, after the shamans sang to him. As he sat down, he looked up and saw me diffuse into a wisp of air, virtually invisible. Instead of my body, he saw a white geometric symbol floating in its place. He whispered to me about what he saw. I looked down. Although it was dark, I could still see myself. Weird.

During another ceremony, I got a sense of how the bobinsana protected the ceremonial space. In my visions, I saw the bobinsana plants neatly situated around the maloka. I looked at their powder-puff flowers. My attention was drawn to their fiber-optic-like appearance. These flowers are made up of many fiber-like stamens that start white and then blend into pink and red at the ends. In my visions, from each bobinsana, red and white streamers shot up high over the center of the maloka, flowing ribbons of energy. These streamers of energy, like ribbons around a maypole, wove themselves into a colorful shield that protected us inside.

On a different night, towards the end of ceremony, I stepped outside for a breath of fresh air. Stepping down from the maloka entrance, I looked for a place to sit down. Just inside of the ring of bobinsanas, the staff had built a few wooden benches. Usually, there are also a couple of wooden chairs out there, primarily for the guards, so they can sit and watch over the ceremony.

At this particular moment, the guards were checking on something over by the entrance to the center, about 150 meters away. I sat down in one of the deep wooden chairs, just to relax and look up at the Milky Way. It was a cool night, almost no bugs. I was alone. Late as it was, the maloka was quiet and so was the forest.

After about ten minutes or so, sitting there, relaxing, I heard someone blowing. After an icaro, sometimes the shamans will blow over the person, a kind of breathy whistle to seal in the icaro. Maybe it was that. Or maybe someone was blowing mapacho smoke over someone to clear energy or offer protection. I wasn't sure where it was coming from, but someone was blowing, *soplando*, shamanically. One smooth blow, no melody or music. Not too loud or forceful, but I could hear it. At first, I thought it was Cvita. It sounded like her *soplo*. I thought she might still quietly be working on someone.

I didn't think much of it. I just sat back and stared into the starry night. Then, as my mind drifted to something else, I heard it again, this breathy blow. I sat up. This time, it sounded like it was coming from outside.

Again, I ignored it and relaxed. I looked over and saw the guards in the distance strolling around with their flashlights. Then I heard it again. "Is that even there?" I thought. "What is that? Am I imagining that?" It happened again. Each time, it faded away, and as soon as I forgot about it, I heard it again. It was as if something were trying to reach me between the lines of my perception. It was not coming from inside. I got the feeling that this *soplo* was for me. If it wasn't coming from the maloka, where was it coming from? Strange.

Then I heard it again. This time it was definitely coming from right nearby. I turned to face it and realized I was looking directly at the bobinsana nearest me. It happened again; it was blowing on me. Crazy as that sounds . . . and I was still coming down from the ayahuasca . . . that bobinsana was blowing right on me. I felt its energy and, for a short while, I communed with this plant. We shared a moment or two, conscious of one another.

Shortly afterwards, I saw that the guard was making his way back to the maloka. The moment had passed. In my heart, I paid my respects to the plant and got up out of the chair. I greeted the guard and then decided to go back into the maloka and share what had happened. Ricardo and the shamans, although happy for me, seemed completely unsurprised. Perhaps on another night, my experience might have stirred more discussion. But that night, it seemed they were more interested in getting some rest. I lay back on my mat, quietly smoked a mapacho, and reflected on what felt like a blessing.

During my bobinsana diet, my dreams would sometimes mix with my ayahuasca visions. In Shipibo tradition, ayahuasca visions are said to access the mystical realm of our dreams. The vision world and the dream world become connected. When our dreams open up, so do our ayahuasca visions. One night, I had a strange dream of being in a large and complicated building, something like an airport. There were many escalators and elevators and lots of people hustling and bustling around. I was on some kind of mission. Apparently, I was to follow a series of nonsensical directions that were somehow being transmitted to my intuition. Following the feeling, I had to go from this floor to that floor, up and then down, over there, and back over here, in the hopes of finding some package that was waiting for me. It was all very confusing until, finally, I found the escalator to the top floor.

This long escalator carried me up and away from all the action, to a rather serene space on the top floor. It was a quiet place, very spacious, and there was a large white desk. Someone was waiting for me at this desk. "Oh, there you are, here's your package," he said. I opened this brown-paper package and found two items inside. One was a thick, rectangular piece of glass, printer paper-size, but about three centimeters thick. A number of intricate designs were etched into it, connecting three embedded convex lenses. It was some kind of magical looking glass, with different lenses, something you could hold up and look through. It appeared to be something that could help me to "see" better in ceremony.

The other item was a shimmering, metallic hand fan, closed. It seemed to be some form of protection, a silver shield that could be opened and closed. It reminded me of something I had seen in the movie *Big Trouble in Little China*. In this film, in a crucial moment, the wizard Egg Shen springs open his metallic fan to deflect some kind of electrical energy attack. This item also seemed useful. These were the two items presented to me in the dream, the magical looking glass and the silver fan.

Ricardo and the shamans had told me how the plants sometimes present you with spiritual gifts in your dreams. The idea is that you will then be able to use these gifts in your shamanic work. The next step was to find these items in my ayahuasca visions.

One night, in ceremony, I did see the magical looking glass—unfortunately, only after I realized that someone had taken it from me. Some dark spirits, wearing hooded trench coats and gas masks, had snatched it from around me and run off down some dark alley. I had to chase them down and forcefully recover it. Once in a while, I conjured up the fan too, but that's probably just my imagination, or maybe not. Things can get tricky in the shamanic realms. Over time, I learned more and more about how to take better care of myself and the energies I was gaining. Some gifts are for sharing and others are best kept to oneself.

# The Song Follows the Vision

Toward the end of the diet, I developed a new icaro, with a new rhythmic melody built around the phrase, *"bobinsana medicina, bobinsana invisible, bobinsana medico"* (medicine of the bobinsana, invisible bobinsana, doctor of the bobinsana). Once again, this icaro had started as a simple tune in the back of my mind. Over the course of the three-month diet, it developed into a song. I really like this song and the way it feels.

Ricardo had taught me that the icaro should follow the vision, the song follows the vision. In our tradition, the icaro is an improvisation. The icaro's lyrics, which might also include a few set phrases, tell the story of what you are doing as you are doing it. The icaro is the medicine that you "are doing."

Shamans do not always have strong visions, and in those times, their song will follow their intuition. Through the training, though, one strives for a more consistent connection to the visions. You want to see what you are doing. For me, the looking glass represented an opportunity to "see" more. When you can "see" the patient's energies in front of you, you can watch as you work. After the bobinsana diet, my shamanic vision improved.

Shortly after the diet, a Colombian-American woman in her fifties came to visit us as a *pasajera*. She was from New York. None of my close family members had been able to visit the center, and so I felt a sort of familial bond with her as a fellow Colombian-American.

She was not really a believer in shamanic medicine. She had come to the center for more of a vague exploration. She had hoped for personal healing but was skeptical, not wholeheartedly on the ayahuasca train. She was shy about drinking the tea and requested smaller doses. At these doses, her experiences were quite mild, and she preferred to keep it that way. As she told me, she was just happy to go through the diet and learn about the ceremony.

After my diet, I wanted to practice my singing. Ricardo had given me permission to practice on the *pasajeros*. One night in ceremony I had some time to myself and decided to walk over to my Colombian friend. I sat down in front of her mat. Ricardo and the shamans were singing to prepare themselves and clear the maloka. Quietly, I asked her how she was doing. Per usual, she said she wasn't really feeling much, not from the ayahuasca nor from the icaros. I asked her if perhaps she wanted to drink more, to amplify her experience. She declined. Then I asked her if it would be all right if I tried singing to her. She said okay.

We had talked earlier about her intentions for that ceremony, and she had said only that she was interested in something broad, like, "letting go of the past and opening my heart." I did my best to sing to her about what she had asked. With my limited Shipibo vocabulary, and a few Spanish words, I sang to her and tried to go through the process of cleaning and opening her heart.

At the time, I was, as we say, "*cantando sin vision*" (singing without visions). Following my intuition, I tried to invoke the plant medicine energies and channel them through my voice. If you are going to follow your intuition, you have to believe in what you are doing. I was just a beginner, and inside, I was filled with doubt. The one thing I could see clearly, even in the dark, was that she was not really into my song.

I finished the song and checked in with her. She was unmoved.

"Did you feel anything from the song?" I whispered.

"No, not really," she whispered back.

Not exactly a confidence builder. Although I comforted myself with the thought that she was, in general, unimpressed with the whole Nihue Rao experience, I was still disappointed. I knew I was just a novice, but it was hard to let it go. I really wanted to reach this woman somehow.

I decided to push things further. Dismissing my feelings of inadequacy, I asked her if she had seen or felt anything at all at any point in the ceremony, before, during, or after the song, *anything at all* . . .

Reluctantly, she mentioned that she had noticed a green energy covering the right side of her face. The energy seemed to extend from her cheek to her forehead and to the side of her scalp. She mentioned that this energy felt negative and that she had a headache on that side.

The rest of the ceremony was still going on and the shamans were still singing. Quietly, I continued to investigate. Sometimes the ayahuasca causes pain while healing a particular area. I asked her where she felt the headache. In the dark, she pulled my hand over her scalp and showed me the spot. She guided my fingers to feel a small dent in her skull. I asked her if she had ever been injured in that spot. She then told me that as a child, back home in Colombia, she had fallen off of a horse and was kicked, there on the right side of her head, hence, the dent.

I suggested that the green energy was probably emanating from this dent in her skull and from the associated trauma. "Maybe," she replied.

"Okay, let me try again, let me try to sing to that," I said. She agreed to a second song.

I started to sing, and as I sang, with my eyes closed, I looked into her face and scalp at the area she had indicated. Ricardo advises seeing with your eyes open, but I usually "see" more with my eyes closed. I saw something, maybe it was just my imagination or my projection, but, in my mind's eye, I saw a green energy over her right scalp and face, mixed with a sort of dark haze. If it was just my imagination, well, that was just fine with me. I was going to imagine cleaning it.

I began to sing to this green energy, about clearing and cleaning it off of her face and scalp. Through the icaro, I called upon the healing energy of the plants to guide my voice and vibration. I also sang to clear and clean the trauma energy from her skull, and from her mind and soul. I sang to cleanse the traumatic memory of the experience and the subsequent fear and suffering. As I continued the song, I saw the green, hazy energy fade.

Once the green energy cleared, I could see the "root" of the problem. At the base of the dent, I could see what looked like a small cluster of pearls. On closer inspection, I could see that this sphere was actually a small cluster of living cells, like those that form from a dividing cell. Through the icaro, I tried to uproot this cluster. Carefully, I detached it and lifted it up. Then, invoking the cleansing energies of water and light, I tried washing it away. I continued clearing and cleaning until it was gone. Then, underneath, at the base of the dent, I saw a small hole in her skull. I then sang to heal and seal this hole. As it closed, I saw her scalp and head began to glow with a golden aura. In my visions, her scalp became smooth. Things settled and it was time to finish the icaro. I closed the song with a quiet *soplo*.

I leaned over and quietly asked her how she was doing. She said she did not feel too much from the song, but she did notice that her headache was gone. She was happy about that, and so was I.

That was the first time that I could see what I was doing during an icaro. My song had followed my vision and, in this case, had also felt more effective. Despite doubts in my mind, I believed in what I was doing. I would need to diet more to open my vision further (and still do), but at least I was getting somewhere. I felt gratitude for the bobinsana, for the medicine, the song, and the protection.

The Colombian woman left a few days later. I haven't had a chance to follow up with her, but I will always be grateful for her patience and her skepticism. Shamanic healing requires trust. By addressing her more immediate concern, the headache, I was able to connect with her. I would then have to rely on a mix of faith, imagination, and my own patience.

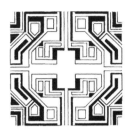

# CHAPTER 19

# Lisa's Migraine Headaches and the Black Dragon

You will not be punished for your anger; you will be punished by your anger.

—Buddha

Further down the road, we were visited by Lisa, a professional dancer in her early thirties from the Southwestern United States. Lisa wanted help with her migraine headaches. Most of us know someone who suffers from this problem; in the United States approximately 15 percent of people are affected.[1] Migraine headaches are generally described as moderate to severe recurrent headaches, typically affecting one side of the head, and lasting anywhere from hours to days. They are often accompanied by nausea, vomiting, and hypersensitivity to light, sound, and sometimes smell.

We are not clear about what causes migraines, but a combination of genetic and environmental factors (once again) is thought to be involved, generating a problem in the nerves and blood vessels of the brain. Migraines are often associated with changing hormone levels, and many women are more affected during their menstrual cycle.

In Lisa's case, she had struggled with menstrual problems for years. As she told me, "Yeah, I've always had problems in that area, as far as irregularity and really bad hormone imbalance . . . Anyways, I used to get [migraines] multiple times a month. That was when I was in my early twenties. When I was twenty-seven, I started getting them like clockwork. The day before my period they would start, and then continue into the first day of my period. It would incapacitate me. I couldn't work. I couldn't do anything."

At the doctor's office, we typically recommend nonsteroidal anti-inflammatories (NSAIDs) like ibuprofen as first-line treatment for migraines and sometimes prescribe additional medications for nausea. Patients are advised to avoid their migraine triggers: certain foods, fatigue, stress, etc., that have brought on headaches in the past. There are also more specific medications for migraine headaches: the ergotamines (found in medications like Cafergot and Migergot) and triptans (including sumatriptan, commonly prescribed as Imitrex), which are, interestingly enough, very closely related biochemically to the psychedelic medicines.[2] LSD is also an ergotamine, and triptans are very closely related to DMT. (In some cases, none of these medications are sufficient, and patients end up being treated with opioid medications for pain.)

Lisa had been taking sumatriptan for her migraines. Typically, for those first two days of her cycle, she would need to take 100 mg of Imitrex (the higher common dose), just to get by. (Although other medications are sometimes also used to prevent attacks, Lisa chose not to be on any preventive treatment.)

I am not a migraine expert, but I had been noticing a pattern among some of the migraine sufferers visiting the center. In talking with them and spending time with them, I observed that several of them had been exposed to a lot of aggression and yelling as children. It was as if their young nervous systems had been overwhelmed by excessive voltage. Some researchers are now supporting the theory that migraines are caused by repetitive stress exposure in childhood.[3-5] As previously discussed, repeated stress exposure can damage the emotional body and stress-response system. Such stress-related damage (accumulated allostatic load) causes a maladaptive stress response. In the case of migraines, this manifests as a dysfunctional response to certain triggers. The brain responds abnormally to certain environmental conditions (psychological and/or physiological), such as certain foods, fatigue, excessive stress, hormonal changes, etc.[1,6]

I asked Lisa if she had been exposed to a lot of aggression as a child. She told me that her father had been very verbally abusive. She said, "He was never, ever physically abusive in any way. [But he] was very verbally abusive. The thing is, my mom used to say, 'When he's good, he's really good. When he's bad, he's horrible.' I have great memories, going to the park, playing with the dogs. [And, I have not-so-great memories.]

"For the first half of my childhood, he and my mom tried to make it work . . . then they would fight. They would have these massive fights. That was bad. Every holiday he was . . . he turns into a rabid dog. He screams and he would toss things off the table. [One time] he shoved the whole Thanksgiving dinner off the table, that kind of insane behavior.

"I, luckily, got left behind [when he would take my brother on trips]. He would refer to me as the girl child: 'The girl child can't come with me to the boy thing,' and he would take my brother. I used to be really sad about that. I would feel neglected and stuff. I'm thankful today because [I learned that] he would take my brother and mess with his head. He's very manipulative. I don't even know the extent of what he said and did to my brother. I know he never hit him or anything, but psychologically he was [relentless].

"My parents actually didn't get divorced until I was eighteen, which is crazy because they totally separated and stopped talking when I was about twelve. [My dad] had his own house. I think that they realized the fighting just got [to be too much]. He would still come over like at Christmas and stuff and they would still have those huge fights, so I don't really know what they were thinking.

"The majority of what happened with me was when I was a teenager. He started getting just nasty with me and saying things . . . put downs. He would put me down all the time. Tell me I was going to end up as trailer trash. Talk bad about my dancing. Just putting me down all the time."

## TAPM Treatment

In 2014, Lisa travelled to the center with her husband, her brother, and his girlfriend. One sunny Sunday afternoon, Lisa and her group roared into the property on a couple of mototaxis. Not long after arriving in the jungle, right after her vomitive, Lisa suffered a terrible migraine.

"That was the worst one of my life, I mean of my entire life. It was brutal."

Ayahuasca and the diet process often stir up pain in problem areas of the body, sometimes even before any of the treatments begin. Maybe it was simply the change of environment, or the travel, but for Lisa, this intense headache was a strange surprise.

Despite her discomfort, she decided to maintain her *vegetalista* diet and go through this severe headache without medication. As tough as this was, she was deeply committed to the process. Sometime later, the terrible headache subsided. Along with the other new arrivals, she consulted with Ricardo and expressed her intentions. (He assigned her the master plant ojé.) The following night, Lisa entered her first ayahuasca ceremony.

I was away from the center at the time and did not arrive until after her first ceremony. While I was away, my cousin Francisco Villegas had come from Colombia to assist at the center.

"The first ceremony was the one that totally knocked me on my [rear]," Lisa recalled. She told me that someone (Francisco) had to keep her from flailing out and disturbing the people around her. In that wild ceremony, she started a deep cleaning process, which involved working through the trauma that she had endured from her father—the anger, the frustration, and the hurt. When I arrived the next day, Francisco let me know that it had been a rough night. Lisa had been a handful, out of control through much of the ceremony.

"Time to lower the dose," I thought.

The following night I entered ceremony with Lisa, Francisco, and the others. She was given less ayahuasca, but was still strongly affected. Sometime after the shamans began singing, on her way back from the bathroom, she just plopped herself down in the middle of the maloka, swaying and moaning quietly. I walked over with Francisco to see what could be done. We needed to try to get her back to her mat, out of the way, but she was deep in the *mareación*. She did not respond to any of our questions.

From the outside, it was hard to know what she was going through. Later she informed me, "I remember I was dealing with a lot of stuff with my dad. I just want to reiterate that a lot of times were good and a lot were bad. It was a constant struggle between feeling loved and feeling rejected, so it caused us to have to try really hard for approval. I was always doing what I could to make him love us, so I think that's where the anger and migraines came from . . . and as a result I carried a lot of guilt from my behavior . . . I feel like my migraines are connected to my cycle but I also think they are connected to all this stuff I was carrying for so long."

As she went through her process in the middle of the maloka, I realized we were not going to be able to move her. "If you can't beat 'em, join 'em," I thought. I sat down on the wooden floor next to her and started singing, trying to bring her back down with my icaro. I tried to center her and help her through whatever she was going through, hoping, if at all possible, to get her back to her mat.

As I sang to her, I started to see something. I saw a thick, beaded strand floating in front of me. It was her DNA, but it was not just her DNA, it was her chromatin. Chromatin is basically the DNA in its protein packaging. The human DNA strand is approximately three meters long. In order to fit neatly into each and every one of our thirty trillion cells, this strand must be magically bundled into each cell nucleus, wrapped tightly around proteins known as histones.

In my visions, this beaded strand of chromatin (made up of DNA wrapped around histones) was glowing pink, and between the beads were little nooks, crannies, and channels. I saw something cruise through one of those narrow channels. It was a long, black dragon swimming laps through the intimate spaces between the beads, round and round the genetic material. As I watched this dragon cruise through the chromatin, I received the message that Lisa's problem was not in her genes (not exactly), but over them. Her migraines were linked to this thin, dark dragon. The song follows the vision, and as I watched I shifted my focus to cleaning out this dragon energy.

This vision reminded me of what I had learned about epigenetics, which is, in a sense, the study of that which exists *upon* the genes. Epigenetics is the study of trait variations that result from external or environmental factors that switch genes on and off and affect how cells express genes. For example, epigenetics explores how external factors like diet and lifestyle can affect the expression of genes causing problems like diabetes, cancer, and Parkinson's disease. Epigenetics, among other things, examines how external factors (like nutrition and pharmaceuticals) alter the surface of the packaging proteins (histones) that the DNA is wrapped around. External factors mark or tag these histone proteins and affect the way their associated segment of DNA strand can be expressed. Like a swimming dragon, these tags reside over the genes and influence them energetically. In general, epigenetics is the study of the way environmental factors (from outside the body and within the body) interact with genes.

Ayahuasca was showing me that Lisa's problem was not genetic, it was epigenetic. Although there may have been others in her family line with migraines, her problem was not fatally locked into her so-called genetic destiny. Her migraines were not caused by a hardware problem, they were caused by a software problem. Lisa's problem appeared to be related to some kind of epigenetic programming problem, maladaptive tagging, if you will. This little dragon represented the unhealthy program. Repeated stress had left her with maladaptive software.

Lisa was not alone in this, of course. Researchers are now investigating the ways in which childhood maltreatment alters epigenetics and leads to migraine headaches later in life.[5,7,8] Epigenetics is a big deal, and I'll get more into this topic in the next chapter.

Sitting there with Lisa, I continued singing to her to try and clear the little black dragon out of the pink-beaded strand of chromatin. I sang to her for a good while, trying to clean and doing my best to center her mind and senses. Eventually, when I felt that I had done enough, I stopped. Lisa was able to speak with me then. She said she was doing slightly better.

I then brought her over to the Shipibo shamans for further treatment, after which my cousin guided her back to her mat in the maloka.

"Someone put me back on my mat. I was a deflated shell. You know what I mean, just deflated. I feel like I released so much that night, and I think that's why the migraine came on."

After her personal icaros, Lisa got another migraine. It was not severe, but it lingered on throughout the ceremony and into the morning, then dissipated. She chalked up this second headache to her healing process. She did feel that the treatment was working on her brain, despite the discomfort. She continued steadfast, with the diet and the ayahuasca ceremonies.

She later told me, "It's like every ceremony, even if I wasn't focused on my dad, I had experiences around it. I would see him and I felt forgiveness and compassion. Every night a little a bit. I don't know what migraines are caused by, but releasing [my anger and guilt], that was a huge thing."

During her fourth ceremony, later in the night, I went over to visit her. She had already received a song from one of the Shipibo shamans and was doing reasonably well. I sat at the foot of her mat and asked if I could sing to her. She said yes and then I sang to her about her trauma and her father, about forgiveness and releasing anger. As I sang, I tried to gather all of the negative energies that I could see and lift them up and out of her. Dark streaks released from her body and began gathering around her head. As I sang further, these dark and hectic energies coalesced into an angry thunderstorm. Sparks of lightning momentarily illuminated its shadows. It covered her entire head.

I sang more intensely, trying to lift these ominous clouds up and away. Working harder and harder, I began to sweat. Slowly the dark clouds rose. I could now see her face, which looked brighter and more clear. I pushed harder, working to send the storm away, far away, asking for assistance from the plants and from divine light. The storm continued to rise off of her head. Motivated by the apparent progress, I kept going and going, until finally something broke loose. Something released and the dark clouds floated away. I sang a bit longer to try and secure this change.

After the song, I asked her how she was doing. She told me she was feeling good and that she had seen a dark cloud over and around her head, like a thunderstorm. During the song, she also felt an intense pressure in her head. Then, as the song continued, this storm rose up over her head, taking the pressure with it.

That was a shocker. I had not yet said anything about what I had seen. That was the first time I shared a vision with the person to whom I was singing. Both of us were describing the energies in the same way and we were both quite surprised. We spoke quietly for a few minutes, exchanging notes about this curious phenomenon. I then excused myself and headed back over to my spot in the maloka.

After the song, Lisa later told me, she felt the pressure and the storm still lingering over her head. Then it floated back down. She once again felt the pressure and started to have a mild migraine. The next day, however, it was gone, and she felt like something had shifted. As she told me, "It was a mix of letting go of all that stuff with my dad and the physical experience of it being taken away."

Throughout the process, the shamans did their best to clean out her energy body, and Lisa herself did her part to release her anger and guilt through forgiveness. After her sixth ceremony, she closed her diet. After a ten-day stay with us, she went home and did not have another migraine for a full year.

When we reviewed her progress about two years after her first visit, in 2016, Lisa told me that after about a year, she did once again have a few headaches; however, they were infrequent and mild. As she put it, "Maybe once every few months. Maybe. For instance, I haven't had one for the last three months. I'm due to start my period tomorrow and I don't have one. [Back before my visit] I would've had one today, so I probably won't get one this month.

"They're so mild that sometimes if I, it's really weird, but if I run and I can get my endorphins going, I can kick them. I used to not be able to do that. [Looking back], my doctor prescribed me six Imitrex pills and now after two years there's only one gone. I took half a pill one time and half another. That's a really big deal.

"You know, I left Nihue Rao feeling more peaceful than I've ever felt in my life. All of my 'issues' seemed to melt away and were replaced with such strong feelings of gratitude for my life and my circle of support. I felt like every challenge in my life was suddenly easy to navigate through. Like I had been given the proper tools for the first time. That being said, I was very surprised by the feelings I got upon returning to the hustle and bustle of the day-to-day. Within the first few days I was super aggravated, and so aware of it. Like I was extra sensitive to the sounds and rush of everyday life, and I just wanted to go back to Nihue Rao. Anyway, over time I've realized that's natural.

"I came home really, really open and all my walls came down. I had totally forgiven my dad. You know the main focus of three of my ceremonies was my anger with my dad. When I came back home, I was full of forgiveness and compassion for him and ready to come to peace with our relationship, so I called him for the first time in two years, and what I got tore me down. He was the same verbally abusive, hateful, terrorizing person I knew he was, but for some reason, I let my guard down, so it hit me very deeply. I had unrealistic expectations that if I came to him from a place of love and forgiveness, that he would respond differently. I was very, very wrong though. I became an emotional wreck and was feeling so defeated.

"At my lowest moment I called [my brother] and told him how stupid I felt and that all the forgiveness had been for nothing because I was still clearly angry. And he said, 'Lisa, if you hadn't gone through what you did, you would never have made the step to call him, and learn what you did today. This is all part of the plan. It is still working.' And he was right. I had idealized what our relationship is, and because I found compassion for him, I made the call, and now, I can see more clearly than ever who he is and always will be. It's all part of a long process, but I know now [that] I'm moving forward in the process, whereas before I was so clouded with anger I couldn't move."

Lisa and some of the members of her group got along well with my cousin Francisco, and they all decided to stay in touch. After working with us, Francisco started doing integration work remotely with Lisa and some of the other *pasajeros* that had been through Nihue Rao.

"Thankfully, Francisco and I had kind of kept in touch and he was starting his life-coaching business. I feel like it all really happened like it should have because I called [Francisco], and that last sh*t storm [my dad] had put on me had to happen for me to go, 'Okay, I can't just come back and expect to be healed. I need to integrate it.' I feel like maybe if I hadn't integrated that and continued to heal and everything, my migraines might've come back. Then within a couple months of talking with Francisco (and this is fully due to ayahuasca), one day I woke up, and the heaviness I [had] felt my whole life was gone, and it's never come back. I used to cry, you probably remember, I used to cry even just [mentioning] my dad. Now it's like I kind of just laugh, because I have totally accepted who he is."

She continues to communicate with her father, who she now realizes is still struggling with his own past. "He doesn't like to talk on the phone anymore, so we just email him. You'll either get the most loving email telling you he misses you and he wants you to come visit, or you'll get an email telling you you're a piece of sh*t. That used to kill me inside. I wouldn't even open the email. Now, I respond to every email with, 'I'm sorry you feel that way, but I'm here when you want to talk.'

"I used to just feel resentful, but now I feel like I've accepted that he's messed up, I'm never going to expect to have a happy father-daughter relationship. It is what it is. I have totally accepted it. Today might be great and tomorrow might not be. Working through my issues with my dad, forgiving him and accepting him, I think that's what helped me get rid of migraines the most.

"I learned to be much more aware of my thoughts and more forgiving of myself. I'm learning every day that inner peace is a practice. I need to practice coming back to myself every single day."

Lisa returned to Nihue Rao in spring of 2016. Her headaches had improved dramatically but she was still struggling with severe menstrual cramps. She returned to continue healing work at the center for two weeks and was placed on a diet of piñon blanco. During the ceremonies, oddly enough she experienced several migraines. She again felt that these headaches were part of her healing process.

I followed up with her two months after her second stay. She told me that she was feeling great, saying, "I am more in control of my emotions than I've ever been. I feel a new sense of calm that I've never had. Also . . . while I was there I had a feeling [that the medicine] was working on those menstrual problems I was having, and I recently had my cycle with barely any cramps. Almost zero pain. I think I talked to you about this before, but my cycles had gotten to a point where I was passing out from the pain, so to have a period with barely any pain is unbelievable to me.

"Also, most of my ceremonies involved self-love in some way and showed me how important that is for me personally, and I have actually surprised myself since I've returned with how much more I trust myself. When I come up against something that would typically have made me panic or go into stress and anxiety mode, I'm finding that my brain is very clear. I'm not automatically emotional anymore. I am certain it is because of the work [the ayahuasca] does on our neural pathways. The changes have been extraordinary so far." So far, she has not had any further migraines.

Migraines, like chronic cough and psoriasis, are thought to be caused in part by neurogenic inflammation.[6,8] Neurogenic inflammation, once again, is inflammation generated by the emotional body, the autonomic nervous system, and the larger PNEI network. It is, in many cases, part of a maladaptive stress response related to the body's ongoing struggle to deal with unresolved emotional trauma. In the cases we have discussed so far (Colleen, Sharon, and Lisa), symptoms associated with this neurogenic inflammation have all been related to unresolved emotional issues. Once these issues were properly addressed, associated skin, lung, and brain symptoms improved. Menstrual problems are in many cases also related to disturbances in the emotional body.

Unresolved emotional issues hang on in the emotional body as what in Shipibo terms would be described as unhealthy energies. These unhealthy energies open one to further energetic contamination. Ricardo may have said something like we need to clean out the spirits or energies associated with Lisa's father's anger. In the visions, these energies appeared to me as a little black dragon and a raging storm. In the physical dimension, under the microscope, these energies manifest as stress-related damage in the stress-response system and larger PNEI network (the emotional body).

These disturbances in the emotional body generate psychosomatic symptoms through processes like neurogenic inflammation. I refer to the stress-related damage underlying these disturbances as allostatic load. Shamanic medicine can be useful in clearing this heavy load, the burden of our accumulated traumas.

How does shamanic medicine interact with the physical body? How can songs and forgiveness dampen neurogenic inflammation? How can plants and rituals affect the physical realms of the brain, nerves, immune system, and hormones? I'd suggest it's through the healing of maladaptive epigenetic programming.

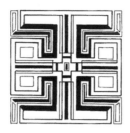

# CHAPTER 20

# Epigenetics, Inheritable Stresses, and Release through Spiritual Healing

. . . I began searching for common ground between indigenous knowledge and Western science, and ended up finding links between shamanism and molecular biology. In the book *The Cosmic Serpent*, I presented the hypothesis that shamans take their consciousness down to the molecular level and gain access in their visions to information related to DNA, which they call "animate essences," or "spirits."

—Jeremy Narby PhD, *Intelligence in Nature*

R
icardo and the Shipibo shamans diagnosed Lisa's migraine problem as an energetic problem, a spiritual problem. In order for Lisa to heal, three things would need to happen: 1) she would need to be cleansed spiritually of problematic energies, 2) she would need to reconcile and transform, through forgiveness, her difficult memories and prior experiences, and 3) she would need

to find a way to love and accept her father. Russ, Colleen, Maria, Karl, and Mike all went through similar healing processes—involving spiritual cleansing, reconciliation, love, and acceptance—and, over time, they also experienced improvements in both their emotional and physical health.

In ayahuasca ceremony, Shipibo shamans approach the healing of the emotional body energetically, directing their attention to cleaning out perceived energetic disturbances, also referred to as negative spirits. In concert with the participant's ongoing personal work, this shamanic cleansing promotes healing in the emotional body and its physical manifestation, the PNEI network.

Lisa needed to be cleansed of the problem energies linked to her past traumas, energies like the black dragon and the dark storm. By her own estimation, shamanic cleansing played a key role in her healing and led to lasting improvements in her physical health.

You may wonder how cleansing energies and spirits, like the black dragon, out of the energy body can result in physical transformation? Well, like bad dreams, these perceived energies originate in negative emotional experiences that end up stored in the emotional body (PNEI network). Strong emotional experiences imprint the emotional body and maintain their energetic influence. Just as strong energetic experiences (e.g., a father yelling at his child) can create these imprints, these imprints can similarly be released through energetic release, as in ayahuasca ceremony. Once a negative energy is released, the emotional network gains an opportunity to return to healthier functioning, paving the way for physical healing.

So where do the energies of past traumas live within the emotional body (PNEI network), and how do these imprints form? Or as Jeremy Narby would put it, where do these "animate essences" and "spirits" live at the molecular level?

Some time ago, I saw the science fiction movie *Jupiter Ascending*. Although I can't say I really enjoyed this movie, I did like some of its ideas. In the film, futuristic space vampires wait around for thousands of years, monitoring a large interplanetary population, waiting for a particular DNA code to pop back up again. They are waiting because when this particular DNA code reappears, it will allow for a particular soul (their dear mother) to once again reincarnate (into virtually the same body). The film basically proposes the idea that, in order to be embodied, the soul requires the presence of a specific genetic code. This suggests that DNA is the seat of the soul (the soul being spirit localized within the life span). The genetic code is where the spiritual rubber hits the road. I thought this was an interesting idea. After all, in biology I had learned that every living thing is a DNA-based life-form.

So, if DNA is the seat of the soul, where does the seat of the soul greet the world? Where is the seat of the seat of the soul? Well, our DNA code sits within our epigenetics, the molecular machinery that exists around and upon the genes (*epi* means "upon" in Greek). This molecular machinery can also be referred to as the epigenome, just as the totality of human DNA can be referred to as the human genome. Thus, the epigenome is the seat of the seat of the soul, acting as the soul's ambassador to this physical dimension. The soul interacts with its physical environment biochemically at the epigenetic level. Spiritual healing interacts with biochemistry at the epigenetic level.

The stories of our emotional traumas live on inside of us energetically. Like the black dragon, these "spirits" live on in our epigenetics. In Lisa's case, this "energy" swimming through her epigenome was linked to memories of abuse stored in her emotional body. The stories of our past traumas and their associated energies live on in our epigenome. Interestingly enough, we now know that epigenetic disturbances play a significant role in emotionally rooted health problems, including all of the illnesses we have thus far discussed: PTSD, depression, psoriasis, addiction, and migraines.[1-10]

Shamans use spiritual techniques to clean out energies associated with accumulated emotional trauma. This mystical cleaning process appears to occur through the healing of maladaptive epigenetic programming. Once more, spirit interacts with biochemistry at the epigenetic level.

In one way or another, childhood trauma has played a significant role in most of the cases I have presented thus far. In Maria's case in Chapter 12, for example, we saw how suppressed memories of early abuse subconsciously affected her emotional and physical state for decades. Although her allopathic physicians did not connect the dots between her childhood trauma and her back and knee pain, healing this trauma, ultimately, would be the key to her physical recovery. This involved ceremonial cleaning of her emotional body and resulted in what she referred to as the "healing of her limbic system."

Current research supports the idea that the "energies" of childhood trauma live on within us as imprints in the epigenome. This seat of the seat of the soul is a virtual house of spirits. The epigenome stores emotional memories and, along with them, the stories of our traumas. In monkey and human studies, the biological memory of childhood maltreatment has been linked to epigenetic imprints.[11-15] In monkeys, these lasting epigenetic imprints can be detected later in life in cells and tissues of the emotional body (PNEI network).[14]

As mentioned in the last chapter, researchers are currently investigating the ways in which childhood maltreatment alters epigenetics and leads to migraine headaches later in life.[16,17] Like spirits, these epigenetic imprints can live on inside of us until death, and can even be passed on to the next generation.[18,19]

Some of these emotional imprints can be useful, as they strengthen the system, like those associated with loving and nurturing interactions. Other imprints, in contrast, can be problematic, telling and retelling stories of repetitive stress damage. As mentioned in the last chapter, epigenetic imprints can occur in a number of ways, including the tagging of histone proteins (DNA packaging proteins).[20] These tags, like other epigenetic alterations, affect the way nearby genes are expressed, modulating their activity, turning them for example "on" or "off." I refer to these modulating imprints as epigenetic programs.

These programs are a form of software that subconsciously records emotional events. In response to one's environment, these programs modulate the way genes are expressed. This is how these emotional memory imprints affect our functioning. Strong emotional experiences can, for example, alter epigenetic software controlling the stress response system, and this altered software will change the way we react to emotional events in the future.

Epigenetic programs participate in emotional memory. In a scenario like Lisa's, epigenetic software developed in response to her father's recurrent abusive behavior and over time accumulated in her epigenome. Without sufficient emotional release, resolution, or relief, these stressful programs continue to accumulate and become part of the operating system. Eventually, repetitive stress generates allostatic load, and the system begins to operate in a chronically stressed mode. This is how maladaptive epigenetic software develops and later causes maladaptive stress responses.

Repetitive stress damage, or allostatic *load*, represents the accumulation of problem programs in the epigenetic software. When Ricardo sees a *pasajero* who looks like he is carrying a lot of unresolved emotional trauma, he says, *está muy cargado* (meaning that that person is very loaded down with cargo, i.e., problem energies). In English, I believe we call it emotional baggage.

There are a lot of ways to approach fixing these epigenetic software problems (by altering, for example, the way histone proteins are tagged) through herbs and pharmaceuticals or even through physical detoxification and purification (like a *vegetalista* diet) (Interestingly enough, compounds within the ayahuasca vine have also been shown to pharmacologically alter epigenetic tagging.[21])

In other words, these biological programs can also be altered spiritually. The epigenetics, the seat of the seat of the soul, responds energetically to love and other mystical phenomena. Childhood maltreatment research and associated monkey studies have demonstrated that young primates (humans and monkeys) respond epigenetically to love and also to the lack of love.[14] The lack of love, the ongoing stress of being unloved, overwhelms the emotional bodies of young primates and leaves them with long-lasting maladaptive epigenetic programming. These monkeys suffer with lifelong social problems and have difficulties coping with stress. In the cases we have thus reviewed, we have seen how related maladaptive programs and energies can be reprogrammed by love and by other faculties of the psyche (soul), including compassion, forgiveness, and gratitude.

In addition to love, we also know that the epigenome responds to meditation and associated altered states of consciousness.[22-24] For some time, researchers have been investigating how meditation influences biochemical function. Research done in the 1970s had established that meditation induces a "relaxation response" throughout the body, altering brain activity and the functioning of the emotional body (PNEI network).[22] Recent studies indicate that this "relaxation response" is driven by underlying epigenetic changes.[23,24] In 2014, investigators in Spain demonstrated that expert meditators can, after only one day of intensive meditation, induce rapid epigenetic changes within their bodies, altering the way inflammatory genes are expressed. Although I am unaware of specific research into the epigenetic effects of psychedelic-induced mystical states, I believe that similar mechanisms are involved.[5]

I believe that Shipibo shamanism and related mystical approaches, at least in part, target epigenetic imprints in the emotional body. Ricardo regularly talks about cleaning the energies of emotional trauma, childhood trauma, *in utero* trauma, and ancestral trauma, all of which have been linked to epigenetic imprints.[6,18,25]

In the case of ancestral trauma, we now know that we inherit epigenetic software from our parents, programs accumulated over the course of their lives, from the stories of their lives, and likely from the stories of their parents' lives, and so on. At conception, the mother's egg and father's sperm carry not only maternal and paternal DNA, but also that DNA's surrounding epigenetic programming and machinery (within, for example, the chromatin). These programs carry the experience of multiple generations and affect the way genes function. These programs help to generate what we have come to know as instincts.

A wild mouse living in a natural setting inherits epigenetic programs from its parents. These programs help tune that mouse's genes to its local ecosystem. Such a mouse is born already responsive to certain smells and sounds in its local environment, instinctually aware of nutritious food options and dangerous predators.[26] Although some of their instincts are locked up in their DNA code, others are inherited in their epigenetics. This epigenetic software allows the individual to respond to changing conditions and prepares future generations. In many cases, this improves survival, as in the mouse whose system from birth is tuned to identify gratifying food sources and dangerous threats.

Inherited epigenetics contribute to useful and advantageous instincts, but they can also pass on maladaptive, disadvantageous programs. These problematic programs carry the burden of what is traditionally described as ancestral trauma. Research done in Europe, for example, has demonstrated that the children of concentration camp survivors 1) inherit epigenetic imprints rooted in their parents' concentration camp experiences and 2) are more likely to suffer from stress-related disorders like anxiety.[18] Although this tendency was previously attributed to parenting problems, further analysis has revealed that it correlates to epigenetic imprints established during war-time trauma. Epigenetic tags affecting stress hormone genes were found in both Holocaust survivors and their children, but not in control groups, similar families living outside of Europe.

In a separate example, researchers at Emory University have proven that conditioned stress responses are inheritable in mice.[27] In their study, some poor group of mice was regularly stressed by an electric shock every time they smelled a particular smell. Over time, these mice were conditioned to react to this smell, even in the absence of the electric shock. This conditioning generated an epigenetically programmed stress response which was then passed on (as ancestral trauma) to subsequent generations of mice. The descendants of these mice freak out in response to a smell that they have never encountered in their lives. This epigenetic programming appears to last for a few generations before washing out over time.

In summary, the emotional body is designed to record and respond to gratifying and stressful events in preparation for the future. Associated epigenetic imprints impact the body's function and can even influence future generations. Although such imprints can be useful and advantageous, others lead to maladaptive stress responses. Recurrent, unrelieved stress can lead to inheritable epigenetic diseases, like anxiety disorders.

The good news is that maladaptive programming is a software problem, not a hardware problem. In disorders rooted in emotional trauma or even ancestral trauma, healing is possible. Excess stress damage can be relieved from the epigenetics, and spiritual healing provides multiple avenues for precisely this kind of relief.

Love and acceptance, for example, can help to bring stress-response functioning back down to a healthier baseline. In cases of ancestral trauma, spiritual healing can even heal a bloodline. In the cases we have discussed so far, faculties of the soul, things like self-love, forgiveness, compassion, and gratitude, have all demonstrated their utility in healing maladaptive stress responses. Spiritual healing meets biochemistry at the epigenetic level. Just as the intense energies of emotional trauma imprint the emotional body, powerful energies associated with profound emotional healing also alter epigenetic programming. When it comes to healing the emotional body, love is the original spiritual medicine.

Our epigenetic machinery does appear to respond to metaphysical intervention: love, altered states of consciousness, mystical experiences, and shamanic techniques. By addressing maladaptive epigenetic software, we can change the way genes are expressed and the way the physical body functions. We'll talk about this more when we discuss Nathan's case in Chapter 22, but for now let's get back to the Fellowship and how the plants helped me to identify problem energies.

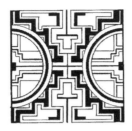

# CHAPTER 21

# Stronger Visions through Further Initiation

Intuition will tell the thinking mind where to look next.

—Jonas Salk MD

During Shipibo shamanic ceremony, in my understanding, the shaman works to clean and clear problem energies associated with maladaptive programming in the emotional body. The *ayahuasquero/a* utilizes ayahuasca to help him or her diagnose and address these problem energies. The ayahuasca shaman advances his or her diagnostic capacity by training with the plants. In my case, the next step in this process was to complete my one year of plant diets under Ricardo and thus my initiation into the practice.

In the fall of 2014, sometime after Lisa's visit, I entered the third segment of my apprenticeship, dieting with ayahuma. Although the *vegetalista* diet can be difficult, over the years I had come to realize that it was as the Shipibos had claimed: dieting master plants is a form of higher education. I wanted to learn more about shamanic healing and clearing problem energies, and Ricardo thought I should diet a "strong tree." He recommended ayahuma. Ayahuma (*Couroupita gui-*

*anensis*) is a tall, tropical tree that grows up to thirty-five meters high and is well known for its large, cannonball-like fruits as well as its large, brightly-colored flowers, blended with pink, red, and purple.

I had heard from Ricardo and others that ayahuma could help open my shamanic vision further and advance my icaros. Like bobinsana, the spirit of ayahuma is also believed to provide protection against malevolent energies and shamanic attack. Ayahuma, however, is considered to be more powerful. A shaman needs protection, first and foremost, to deal with the stronger energies that may present themselves in ceremony, often from one or more of the *pasajeros* (like, for example, Russ's war trauma). And, there are also those times when a shaman must face other difficult energies, energies originating from outside of the ceremony, from nature and the larger world.

Traditionally, Shipibo shamans recognize witchcraft as a potential source of such dark energies. The shaman must learn to protect him- or herself against the ill will of evildoers. I myself am not very interested in witchcraft, but there is no doubt that ayahuasca shamanism has always had its dark side, and some individuals, referred to by some as sorcerers or *brujos* (witches), diet and train with master plants strictly for malignant purposes. Rather than learn about humility, healing, and encouragement, these individuals are more interested in power, destruction, and manipulation. As in business and politics, all is fair in the world of plant shamanism.

Some people, particularly those who have been through major healing experiences, find it hard to believe that ayahuasca could be used for negative purposes. I, however, have learned that nature and the plants are rather neutral when it comes to human affairs. One morning after ceremony, I remember listening to one *pasajero*'s experience of this neutrality. The night before, the ayahuasca had told him that, for humans, life here on earth is largely about free will. For this reason, humans are free to make their own decisions and learn things, if necessary, the hard way. Ayahuasca and the plants can guide you to your heart's feelings and help you to see the damaging effects of your choices, but the master plants will not necessarily get in your way. Ultimately, you are left to your own decisions, for better or worse.

The master plant ayahuma is known for its strong medicine and for its dark side. At Nihue Rao, because of this dark side, ayahuma is dieted only by more advanced practitioners. Master plants like piñon blanco and ojé, which are said to be full of light with little or no dark side, are considered to be better choices for beginners.

The dark energies of the plants, as in the case of ayahuma, are, once again (as mentioned in Chapter 16 in regards to marijuana), called *shitanas* in Shipibo. Instead of teaching spiritual healing, these *shitanas* are believed to teach witchcraft. Although such energies can be useful in self-defense, a healer must be very careful with the *shitanas* he or she collects, as these energies can contaminate one's medicine. In Ricardo's tradition, when one diets a strong plant like ayahuma, one's master follows along throughout the process to help clean the *shitana* energies (in ceremony) and maximize medical education.

I was not too worried about the *shitanas* of ayahuma. I knew that I was clear about my intentions and that Ricardo could help me to, as we say, "keep it in the medicine." I planned to diet for three months to round out my apprenticeship. By that point in the fellowship, I had been involved with ayahuasca for seven years, and for four of those years, I had been deeply involved in ceremonial work at the center.

As I had hoped, my ceremonial experiences became increasingly visionary during the ayahuma diet. During the first week, I had my first introduction to the spirit of this plant. During one ceremony, I was brought inside of a large tree. Inside the hollow of this tree, I found myself seated in a dark space three or four meters in diameter, big enough to look around in. Dark wooden walls arched over me, covered in smoldering red designs. These intricate designs lit up intermittently against their dark background flaring like charcoal. It was kind of scary in there. Was this the medicine of ayahuma or its *shitana?* I wasn't sure. I just sat there respectfully and cautiously. I felt the presence of a large spirit over me but could not see anything beyond the dark walls. Although there was no clear communication, there was a sense of mutual acknowledgment. The glowing designs breathed on. Everything was going to be okay. Even though I felt safe in the protection of this tree, I was also a little uneasy; things were darker than I was used to. I sat there and observed, trying to take in the energy of the slowly pulsing designs, until, eventually, the vision faded.

Sometime later in the diet, ayahuma taught me a few new things. One night, ayahuma showed me how to interact with the visions from a new perspective. During a quiet phase in the ceremony, before Ricardo and the shamans had started singing, I looked out and saw three menacing monsters leering at me. Standing some distance away, they weren't too threatening, but they were in my way, blocking me from getting into something more productive. They just felt like a distraction, and I wanted them to go away. Ayahuma gave me a new strategy. In my mind, I was directed to flatten this unpleasant multidimensional vision down into a two-dimensional screen. Once I had this monster scene in flat screen, I could turn it, rotate it, flip it around, play with it, and eventually discard it. I had never thought of approaching visions like that. Ayahuma was opening my mind to the possibilities.

On a different night, I encountered a more aggressive energy. A menacing, shadowy spirit appeared in my visions. It came close and tried to bother me. Although part of me was happy to be seeing something, I was not in the mood for negative visions. Where was this thing coming from? I was too tired that night and I didn't really care. It kept gesturing at me, trying to threaten me, moving closer. Frustrated and angry, I began to contemplate how I might banish this dark spirit from my ceremonial experience. While I was thinking about burning it or destroying it somehow, suddenly, out of nowhere, gnarled tree branches shot out from behind me and struck this creature with splintering fists. Unbeknownst to me, ayahuma had released a couple of jaw-breaking haymakers in my defense. These brutal branches obliterated the shadowy spirit and it faded away. True, this was exhilarating, but it was also rather shocking. I should have spent more time trying to determine where this spirit was coming from, making sure that it wasn't connected to anyone. But it was too late. It felt out of control. I knew I would have to work further to control my anger, frustration, and impatience. As the diet continued, I worked on these areas. Along the way, little by little, Ricardo helped me to clear out and control the ayahuma *shitana*.

More importantly, I also connected to ayahuma's medicine. During this diet, Ricardo allowed me to continue to practice on the *pasajeros*. Thanks to ayahuma, I was now consistently seeing at least something every time I sang to someone. As with the Colombian woman and Lisa, I had had visionary experiences when singing to others, but this had been more the exception than the rule. Now I was seeing energies and stories in every *pasajero*. (I will describe another one of these interesting visionary experiences below.) I remember telling Ricardo about this exciting shift in my practice. He said something like, "Joe, you would not believe how slow this process is." As he often says, "Getting sick is fast . . . and easy, the dark side is like that, fast and easy. But healing takes time. Learning to become a healer is a very slow process."

Just a week shy of the three months I'd planned on, I had to end my ayahuma diet due to a second bout of malaria, an unfortunate occupational hazard. Having learned from my first experience, I knew that once I started the pharmaceutical treatment. I would recover quickly from the miserable fevers, sweats, and body aches. Before long I was eating normally and feeling better. In the end, it was all well worth it. I completed my basic training as an apprentice and, ever since that three-month ayahuma diet, more often than not, I have visions when I sing icaros to people (even on nights when my experience is not otherwise visual). As promised, the ayahuma diet advanced my practice and strengthened my confidence.

After completing this diet, there was no big party or congratulations, simply the opportunity to keep working and practicing. I was now thinking about running my own ceremonies. At the center, there were a few opportunities to do so on off nights with a few friends, but most of my practice still came during the larger ceremonies under the supervision of Ricardo and the other Shipibo shamans.

As my visions opened, I would sometimes see things in people that they had not told me about. Such visions can be relevant to the healing process, but should be considered carefully. If sharing such visions seems appropriate, they should be treated with some skepticism and then confirmed. Like dreams, the ayahuasca often speaks through metaphor. In the wide world of shamanism, there is plenty of room for projection. We should not be too attached to our own interpretations. Good doctors not only consider what they know (or what they think they know), they think about what they don't know. Respectfully and humbly, one works to find the medicine in such revelations.

Not too long ago, a young man named Larry, in his thirties, visited the center from the East Coast of the United States. During his initial consultation, Larry discussed what he wanted to work on during his two-week stay. Most of all, he wanted to address sexual issues. He had become overly involved with Internet pornography and was simultaneously having problems performing sexually with his live-in girlfriend.

I think most people who were there at the time would agree that Larry is a kind, thoughtful, and good-natured person. His experiences during ayahuasca ceremony were generally very pleasant. They were not, however, very visionary. Regarding his ceremonies, Larry reported that the ayahuasca consistently made him feel very good physically and mentally. Each night, the ayahuasca directed him through a wild series of spontaneous and sometimes involuntary movements of his body and limbs during which, as he put it, he "jammed" to the icaros. His ceremonial experiences were consistently powerful but not at all troubling or difficult. Larry began to get the idea that perhaps he was healthier than he had previously thought.

In the post-ceremonial morning conversations, he was open about what he was trying to work through. He talked about being grateful for his positive ceremonies and attributed these experiences to a generally positive childhood. During his stay, he dieted ajo sacha and was very respectful of the process. And still, there was a part of him that felt like he wasn't learning anything. He continued to be blocked to the visions. In some cases, this can be because one doesn't want to see what the ayahuasca wants you to see. Other times, this block can be due to a lack of interest in a potentially relevant memory or past experience.

One night in ceremony, I wandered over to the foot of his mat to see how Larry was doing. It was a bit later in the night and he was coming down from another positive experience. He had spent most of the night feeling good, squirming around and kicking his legs in the air. I asked him if he had received any information or personal insights. Once again, he had not received any particular knowledge.

I asked if I could sing to him, he said okay, and I started to sing my icaro. In the beginning, as is often the case, I couldn't really see anything. I didn't have a plan for the song. It was hard to know where to begin, but I decided to try and focus on his sexual problems and on opening up his visions, hoping the ayahuasca would reveal something.

I tried to limbically resonate with him, trying to tune in to his internal world, feel into what he feels, and see what that might open up for me. I could see some parallels between us, two seemingly nice guys who are generally pretty open, but who, like most people, keep a few things to themselves. Tuning in to him allowed my intuition to feel into his situation. Ricardo always advises us to protect ourselves when singing and to be careful about how we connect to a *pasajero's* energies. So, careful not to take on Larry's energies, I tuned in and observed.

I continued singing, and then a few minutes later, I noticed something. It was faint at first, but it was there. There was some kind of ghoul quietly hiding out deep inside his chest. I looked it over. As Rolando had once advised me, I did not go right after it. Instead I studied it for a while, trying to understand the story behind the story of this ghoulish spirit. Something was hidden there, and although outward appearances looked good, deep down, something uncomfortable was attached to this ghoul. I thought about leaving it alone, not really sure if I wanted to engage it.

I continued my song with more general themes, trying to clean his mind, heart, and body, trying to open his visions. But there it was, and it wasn't going anywhere. The ayahuasca was letting me know, "You need to deal with this ghoul."

I decided to go after it, trying to dig it out and detach it from his body and soul. I sang to try and untangle this dark spirit from whatever energy it was connected to in his life. Through the icaro, I tried to fish it out, draw it out, and then I saw it more clearly. It was a dimly glowing skull. Larry was initially sitting cross-legged in a near-lotus position, but as I focused in on this skull, Larry raised his knees and put his feet flat down on the mat. (I later asked him why he moved his legs in that moment. He said he just felt uncomfortable and needed to change his position.)

Once Larry was in this new position, the ghoulish skull morphed into the skeleton of a human baby, surrounded by a grey aura. As I sang, this ghoulish baby descended into Larry's abdomen and nestled into the fetal position. Intuitively, I was informed that Larry had participated in an abortion. I could not be sure if this was true, but I received the message that his child had been aborted, and this was the spirit of that dead baby somehow attached to him.

This skeleton continued to descend. Larry's legs were still propped up and the baby slid down. The ghoulish baby birthed out of him energetically and ended up in between his legs in front of me. In the song and in my imagination, I then presented this grey spirit up to the light and prayed for its transcendence, working to clear any other attached darkness. I then kept working until things seemed to clear up.

I eventually finished the song and checked in with him. Something had moved in his experience. At last, he had some visions. He saw a gathering of people and in the distance, barely noticeable, he saw his father. He said, "I remember feeling like everyone was a part of my family (a universal family that spanned millennia) but, through nonverbal communication, my father reaffirmed his position in my life as my father and closest family member." He had a vision about fatherhood. I told him that I wanted to talk to him about what I saw, but that I would do so later, in private.

Later that night, after Ricardo had closed the ceremony, I went over to speak with Larry. His neighbors were off chatting on the other side of the maloka and he was resting alone. I told him that I wanted to tell him about what I had seen but that first I wanted to ask him something. I asked him if he had ever been part of an abortion. He said yes, with a girlfriend from college, but that he had never told anyone else about this.

I then told him about the birthing process that I had observed. Leaving all judgment aside, I let him know that in our experience abortion becomes an energetic problem, a spiritual wound that eventually needs to be addressed and healed. He was surprised to hear this, as he had not previously given the abortion much thought. Larry felt that maybe the ayahuasca was making him go through what his ex-girlfriend had had to go through.

The energies associated with prior abortions often come up during ceremonial healing, primarily in women. In Larry's case, this pregnancy had been an accident, but he admitted that he should have been more careful. Our conversation prompted thoughts of his prior promiscuity, some reckless behavior, and a shame that he had associated with sexuality. This was a real breakthrough for Larry and directed him to start working on reconciling his prior recklessness and clearing the associated shame.

In the shamanic tradition, even spontaneous miscarriages should be addressed. While they may not generate the same feelings of guilt or shame, they still leave behind a spiritual wound and energetic imprints connected to death and trauma. If this energy is not cleaned, it may later manifest as physical illness.

Sometimes we don't know what kind of energies are in the way of our healing and our growth. Ayahuasca and the plants can help us to see what we normally don't see, guiding our intuition. Intuition then tells the thinking mind where to look next. This kind of guidance was crucial in Nathan's case, whom you will read about next. Nathan came to Nihue Rao to address many years of depression and an ongoing struggle with Crohn's disease (an inflammatory bowel disease).

# CHAPTER 22

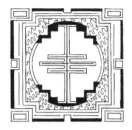

# Nathan's Crohn's Disease

## Mystical Reprogramming
## and the Healing of a Broken Heart

> If you desire healing,
> let yourself fall ill
> let yourself fall ill.
>
> —Rumi

In January 2015, Nathan came to Nihue Rao looking for help. I actually missed most of his stay. I had been back in the States for the holidays, but I did meet him briefly at the end of his visit. Martina, Cvita, and Cvita's husband Markus Drassl (Martina's brother) had all been with Nathan throughout his stay and suggested that I follow his progress. By that time, with my basic shamanic training complete, I focused on my next mission, working to bridge allopathic medicine and traditional shamanism. I had begun stringing together stories for this book and I was looking for interesting cases. I had seen significant improvement occur in a few cases of irritable bowel syndrome (IBS) and inflammatory bowel disease. I was looking to write about one of them, and the team drew my attention to Nathan. After three weeks in Peru, Nathan's longstanding Crohn's disease improved dramatically.

In the spring of 2016, more than one year after his three-week stay at Nihue Rao, I interviewed Nathan about his health and his time in the Amazon. Nathan is a locomotive engineer from Canada who was in his mid-forties when he visited the center. He had suffered from Crohn's disease for most of his life. Crohn's disease is an inflammatory bowel disease (IBD) that causes inflammation in the lining of the gastrointestinal (GI) tract, commonly affecting the colon, or large intestine. This disease causes abdominal pain, severe diarrhea, fatigue, weight loss, and malnutrition. Crohn's disease is thought to be caused by a combination of environmental, immune, and bacterial (gut flora) factors in genetically susceptible individuals.[1] There is no accepted cure for Crohn's disease, however, therapies can greatly reduce its signs and symptoms and even bring about long-term remission.

Nathan's symptoms started when he was an adolescent: intense, recurrent abdominal pain and frequent bouts of diarrhea. He was initially treated with immunosuppressive steroid medications, like prednisone, to calm the inflammation in his guts. He was also treated for pain with opiate medications like Tylenol #3 and Percocet. By age twenty-three, ongoing inflammation had damaged his intestines to the point that he developed a perforation (hole). This perforation transformed into an abnormal connection (fistula) between his intestines and bladder. Urine and stool were then able to pass back and forth freely across this fistula, causing multiple infections.

Nathan became very ill and was hospitalized. He underwent emergency surgery to repair his intestines and bladder. Biopsies taken during the surgery confirmed the diagnosis of Crohn's disease. After the surgery, he recovered. However, despite the severity of his disease, Nathan did not maintain regular follow-up with his doctors. He was struggling with emotional problems and did not like the way immunosuppressive steroids made him feel.

Over the years, Nathan had had further intestinal problems and needed two additional surgeries, each one involving a bowel resection (the removal of a segment of intestines). In this kind of surgery, after a bowel segment is removed, ideally, the remaining healthy "ends" are reconnected as soon as possible (for normal bowel function, i.e., so you can use the toilet normally). However, after one of his surgeries, due to ongoing infection, his intestines could not immediately be reconnected. He was then forced to use an external ileostomy bag for three months, until his bowels could be safely rejoined. In between these surgeries, he was primarily treated with pain medications. Nathan's last bowel resection was in 2010.

From 2010 to 2012, Nathan's digestion improved. But eventually his symptoms returned: recurrent abdominal pain and up to fifteen bowel movements a day, sometimes bloody. Throughout these years, Nathan was not taking very good care of himself. Before coming to Nihue Rao, despite his symptoms, he had never really considered improving his diet, which consisted of a lot of highly processed foods and a daily bacon-filled breakfast sandwich. Nathan had other things to worry about.

Nathan had been depressed for most of his life. Psychological problems like anxiety and depression are common in IBD (inflammatory bowel disease).[2,3] This is theorized to be due to the stressed psyche's influence on the brain-gut axis, the hypothalamic-pituitary-adrenal axis (the HPA axis, i.e., stress-response system) and the peripheral nervous system (the autonomic nervous system).[4] That is to say, Crohn's disease involves disturbances in multiple regions of the emotional body (PNEI network). As with psoriasis and migraine headaches, intestinal inflammation in Crohn's disease has also been correlated to emotional body dysfunction and related neurogenic inflammation.[5,6] As you may have guessed, multiple lines of evidence also indicate that epigenetic disturbances (maladaptive software) play a significant role in the development of Crohn's disease.[7,8]

Despite his chronic depression, Nathan had had only minimal exposure to psychotherapy and psychiatric treatment. Nathan had had a pretty traumatic childhood. He never knew his biological father, and the man who he was led to believe was his father died when he was only five. His mother was involved with some physically abusive men, including the man that became his mother's husband, with whom Nathan lived with from ages six to thirteen. After years of severe physical abuse, at age thirteen, Nathan ran away from home. He stayed briefly at a shelter and then, before long, he started living on his own. He lied about his age, started work, and found a place to live. He had some support from an uncle.

Nathan's digestive problems developed in his adolescence, and as an adult, he was depressed and angry. He told me that he had regularly gotten into problems with people who "challenged me on streets and bars or just wherever, just bad people." In 2001, a former girlfriend asked him to go to therapy to work on his anger, and for some time he went. Therapy helped Nathan to manage his anger.

Despite his problems with anger, Nathan was never physically abusive with his romantic partners. He did, however, struggle in relationships, and his depression often made things worse. After his 2010 surgery, Nathan's mood declined further. His then-wife encouraged him to seek help and get on antidepressants. He tried antidepressants for three months but did not find them helpful. In his own words, "I don't like pills and I don't think they worked anyway. I think they just made things worse."

Nathan did not seek any further help from therapy or psychiatry. He continued to utilize pain medications intermittently and sometimes used edible forms of medical marijuana to calm his guts. Nathan told me that he never developed any serious problems with drugs or alcohol. Over the course of our conversation, he then revealed to me that he had been suicidal for most of his life. Sometime in 2013, his suicidal thoughts became more serious. He began to set dates to end his life.

In 2014, Nathan first heard about ayahuasca while listening to celebrity Joe Rogan's podcast. He heard stories about people going to the Amazon to heal depression. He then learned of Nihue Rao from journalist Amber Lyon's website reset.me. He contacted the center and scheduled his visit.

As I mentioned earlier, Nathan arrived at Nihue Rao in January of 2015. At that time, Ricardo was running the center with Cvita and Markus. Markus, a visual artist by trade (and the creator of this book's cover art and chapter drawings), had also been working and training with us for years. He is a very talented individual who brings a special combination of mental clarity and lightheartedness to his work. As I was working on this chapter, I asked Markus about his assessment of Nathan at the time of his arrival. Markus told me that Nathan was clearly a kind and gentle person, but extremely desperate. During his first days, he was regularly talking about suicide. Nathan had told Markus that Nihue Rao was his last option: if the plants couldn't help him, he didn't want to go on living.

Nathan started his *vegetalista* diet with a *vomitivo*, and after reviewing his situation and intentions with Ricardo, he was prescribed the master plant ojé. As a reminder, the sap of the ojé tree is used traditionally to treat intestinal parasites and is known for its purgative and detoxifying properties. Ricardo hoped that the ojé would help his digestion and spiritually inspire him to see beyond his depression. Once settled into his ojé diet, Nathan started entering ayahuasca ceremonies.

During our 2016 follow-up interview, Nathan told me, "When I showed up there, I was really worried about the bathroom because the day before I arrived, I was still going fifteen times a day. [Once on the diet] it was probably down to about three times on the first day. After the first two ceremonies, which were quite vile at both ends (vomiting and diarrhea), other than the ceremony bathroom breaks, I didn't [really need to use] the washroom at all, except to pee. That was just after the first two ceremonies. I don't really remember feeling any abdominal pain when I was [at the center]. I can't remember any at all. I had stomach pains from puking. But Crohn's pain . . . I can't remember if I had any at all, actually."

The switch to a whole-foods diet of primarily fresh fish and vegetables probably made a big difference for Nathan's digestion. He also likely benefitted from the addition of some jungle bacteria to his gut flora. In Nathan's experience, though, the ojé and the ayahuasca ceremonies played a major role in his intestinal healing, and not just through gastrointestinal purging.

Nathan was an especially visual *pasajero*. He had several "out of this world" mystical experiences. He described a cleansing episode in one of his earlier ceremonies when "snakes are coming after me, and I'm throwing up, I'm in the bathroom, at this time, and I'm puking into the bucket and the snakes are in the bucket, when I would puke in the bucket, the snakes would lick it and then they would die."

In another ceremony, he says, "I saw this bald guy riding on a gold chariot; [at first it was] Jean-Luc Picard from *Star Trek*, then his face morphed into Gandhi, and then it morphed into my doctor, who was bald as well. When my doctor got close, I yawned and he tried to put a pill in my mouth that I refused, and then he turned into this huge viper, so large, and then he took off."

He was particularly impressed by his multiple experiences with extraterrestrials. These strange entities, possibly higher-dimensional beings, were crucial to his healing. In one vision, he was brought aboard their spaceship. There, they were "working on me, fixing, kind of rewiring my brain. The aliens were working on me with a computer."

On the spaceship (in the bathroom at Nihue Rao), he watched as one of the aliens performed this reprogramming. He described this experience to me: "I can hear the hum, it's so loud in my head. It's almost overpowering. And then, he (the alien) would look at me. In the ship, I'm in this glass box to protect the aliens from me, but I'm on the toilet at the same time. The alien was just reprogramming, then he turned around and looked at me with no emotion, just to see the progress that he was making. And then, he'd turn away and I just purged like crazy. And then at one point, it seemed like I was having an out-of-body experience behind the toilet, seeing my hunched over body holding a puke bucket. And then he panicked and hits this button, and I was on the toilet and I felt electricity going up my thigh and I could see something coming up from behind me, bluish-white energy" . . . and then the vision faded.

Nathan also had more personal experiences during his ceremonies. One night, he asked the ayahuasca to show him who his real father is. Nathan told me, "I had a horrible childhood, losing my dad when I was five, supposedly, if he was my dad. Bad stepfathers, and this last one who is still with my mom was horrible to us, violent beatings and stuff, right? Ayahuasca showed me him, this last [stepfather], and said something like, 'Forget about your father, this is your dad.' From age six to thirteen, before I moved out, he was the guy that raised me. Ayahuasca said, 'Just forgive him, and he can be Dad.'"

In another ceremony, Nathan was shown a vision of an aunt molesting him as a child and also molesting some of his cousins. He had had no prior memory of this sexual abuse. At the time, though, this information resonated with him. He knew, however, that he would have to investigate this further when he got back home.

"Another really crazy ceremony was with Cvita," he told me. Cvita had gone over to his mat and asked if she could sing to him, and Nathan said yes. He was in the midst of a very intense and dark ayahuasca experience. Cvita started her icaro. Throughout the song, the ayahuasca gave Nathan clear instructions, first telling him to close his eyes.

"So, I'm sitting cross-legged with my hands on my lap, and Cvita's just singing and singing, and there's lots of snakes and piranhas biting on me at the time. It was a very dark ceremony.

"So now she's singing and it's getting lighter, lighter, and lighter. And then, there were butterflies and dragonflies, very earthy, kind of like a garden sort of thing. And then I got this overwhelming feeling that the song was going to be over right away. When I got that feeling, this huge piranha comes from above her towards me.

"I didn't say anything, or flinch. At that moment, Cvita got up on her knees, like her high knees, and pushed my head down. She pushed my head down and was singing and singing and singing, doing what she does. When my head was down, in my hands, I saw a shape of a heart like a child would draw, but it was broken.

"So then, Cvita grabs my hands and squeezes them together to squeeze this heart together. I then opened my hands and I could see that the heart was fixed, but then it would break again. And she'd close my hands again, squeeze them, open them, and look, it was fixed and then it would break again. So then, she went to my chest and my back and continued singing. And then she looked at my hands again, and the heart was fixed."

Nathan's Crohn's Disease                                    219

Nathan did not at any point communicate verbally with Cvita during the song. "That was the craziest ceremony there, because she was manipulating my hands. It was really strong for me."

After three weeks of ceremonial healing, Nathan completed his ojé diet. He left feeling much better and returned home to Canada. Shortly after getting back, he became ill and was diagnosed with malaria and two gut parasites. For two weeks, he was very sick with frequent diarrhea. A medical doctor treated him with pharmaceutical medications and he improved. Once he recovered from this illness, he noticed that he no longer needed to use the restroom very often.

Once he felt better, he visited his mother and stepfather. He discussed his ceremonial experiences with them. They knew why he had gone to Peru; he had told his mother that he was very depressed and suicidal. Although his mother still had not revealed his biological father's identity, Nathan decided to tell his stepfather about what the ayahuasca had told him. He told him about the vision of his stepfather being his "dad," not his father, but his dad. His stepfather accepted this role and apologized to Nathan for all of the abuse. Nathan recalled, "He said he just wasn't a good dad, he didn't know how to be a dad, he's just a truck driver, he didn't know how to be a dad. We're all good now. It's good." As Nathan says, they have mended all of their fences.

He then investigated the vision about the molestation and spoke with his cousins. They verified the sexual abuse. His aunt had molested Nathan from ages five to twelve and had also sexually abused his cousins during that time. He spoke to their mother about this and his own mother. Nathan's mother wept. She had no idea. He continues to work though his feelings about this abuse, and he continues to forgive.

Since his return from Peru, and following up on his "ayahuasca homework," Nathan's mood has improved. Although he was still going through his divorce at the time we spoke, he told me that he no longer felt depressed. Up through the spring of 2016, he reported that there was really only one day when he felt overwhelmed and helpless, a day when he was in court for his divorce. He and his ex-wife had been battling over custody of their children. These feelings were only fleeting. He recovered quickly and told me that he has otherwise felt positively about his life. He has not had any further suicidal feelings. He avoids stressors that previously aggravated his Crohn's disease, and he is now working toward his next goal: a successful romantic relationship.

After the plant diet, Nathan became, as he says, "a bit" more careful about what he eats. The three-week retreat gave him an opportunity to explore a simpler diet, and now he eats more fresh vegetables, drinks kombucha, and takes daily probiotics. Since his time at Nihue Rao, Nathan has not suffered with abdominal pain. On a bad day, he might need to use the restroom three or four times, at most. Once in a while, he does experience some abdominal cramping which feels like it might develop into diarrhea. When he feels this way, he takes an edible form of medical marijuana. This slows his guts and resolves his symptoms.

His change in diet has likely contributed to the dramatic and prolonged improvement in the level of inflammation in his intestines. In his experience, this decreased inflammation has also paralleled major improvements in his mental health. Deep emotional healing with the plants and associated spiritual techniques shifted something inside of Nathan's body. This mental and physical shift happened after significant energetic purging from his emotional body, mystical reprogramming of his "brain," and the healing of his broken heart. Spiritual healing helped Nathan to find emotional healing. This emotional healing allowed for subsequent healing of his mind-body. Given the nature of depression and Crohn's disease, I assume that some of this healing happened through energetic clearing of maladaptive epigenetic software.

# Nathan's *Susto*

When Nathan was preparing to leave Nihue Rao, the team talked to him about staying longer. There was still a lot more cleaning to do. Like Maria, Nathan had also been diagnosed with *susto*, the indigenous diagnosis for those individuals whose souls have been scared out of their bodies due to a strong shock, fright, or trauma. This is akin to the concept of soul loss, for which the treatment is soul retrieval. Nathan had experienced violent physical abuse and sexual abuse as a young child. This resulted in a disassociated state in which he lost access to repressed memories. As you'll recall, this disassociation disrupts limbic/emotional development. Cross-cultural psychologist Monica Williams has stated that the symptoms of *susto* are actually quite similar to post-traumatic stress disorder (PTSD), which includes anxiety, avoidance, jumpiness, sleep disturbances, and depression.[9]

When we spoke last, although he was feeling better, Nathan was still concerned about this *susto* diagnosis. Ricardo had told him that there was still more work to do. I encouraged him not to worry too much about this and suggested that he simply continue his healing and integration work. When the time is right, I know he will seek further shamanic treatment.

Nathan's case is an impressive example of how spiritual healing techniques can affect inflammatory bowel disease. In medicine, whenever possible, one should go after the root of the problem, the underlying causes. Emotional trauma and childhood maltreatment, including physical and sexual abuse, were the major underlying causes of Nathan's mental and physical illness. Although his diet needed to be addressed, Nathan was also in need of deep emotional healing. Mystical access paved the way to his recovery.

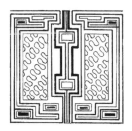

# CHAPTER 23

# Adam's Anxiety and the Calming Power of Compassion

Compassion becomes a bridge to the world outside. Trust and compassion for oneself bring inspiration to dance with life, to communicate with the energies of the world.

—Chogyam Trongpa, *Cutting through Spiritual Materialism*

Don't give in to your fears. If you do, you won't be able to talk to your heart.

—Paulo Coelho, *The Alchemist*

By the time 2015 ended, I had spent half or more of each of five years at Nihue Rao. Life at the center was often beautiful. There was the forest, of course, in a thousand shades of green, the mighty rain, the wonderful people, and the starry, starry nights. And there were the rough times, tough ceremony nights, scary nights, management squabbles, personal dramas, etc. Through the ups and downs, I continued to be inspired by our healing work. In addition to the cases I've presented in this book, I had witnessed hundreds of people go through profound healing experiences at Nihue Rao. Being off the grid and in the forest, however, with limited Internet, it was never easy to keep up with them, to find out how they had fared back home. We were busy enough just caring for the *pasajeros* on site.

By 2016, I had decided to spend more time away from Nihue Rao to work on other projects, follow up with the *pasajeros*, and write this book. The center had become more established, and there was more help available. There was more time to develop my ideas and integrate my experiences as both doctor and shaman.

Nihue Rao was originally Ricardo's vision, and although it had become my home away from home, I started thinking about my own independent path. The Fellowship of the River was changing course, or maybe it was just flowing back into the ocean. In 2016, I decided to reduce my time at the center down to about four months.

While away from Peru, I stayed in communication with the center and helped manage things from afar. I continued to help screen our *pasajeros*, occasionally answering questions online. Early in 2016, while back in Arizona, Martina asked me to respond to a few questions from a fifty-five-year-old man named Adam. Adam was looking for help with his anxiety.

Anxiety disorders occur when people feel frightened, distressed, and uneasy for no apparent reason.[1] So many of us experience anxiety from time to time. According to the National Institutes of Mental Health, a full 18 percent of the U.S. adult population experiences an anxiety disorder each year, with over 22 percent considered severe. There are different kinds of recognized anxiety disorders, including, but not limited to, generalized anxiety disorder, social anxiety disorder, specific phobias, and PTSD. Anxiety disorders, like depression and addiction, have been linked to the same kind of narrow-minded thinking that I discussed in Chapter 5 (associated with overactivity in certain brain regions [Default Mode Network]). This kind of thinking makes it harder to stay in touch with your feelings and the world around you. It disconnects you from your heart. In the case of anxiety, inappropriate fear feeds this disconnection and contributes to further problems in the emotional body. Anxiety disorders involve disturbances in the limbic brain (amygdala), the stress-response system (HPA axis), and the autonomic nervous system (causing, for example, rapid heart rate and high blood pressure).[2]

Anxiety can be caused by drugs (caffeine, alcohol, or benzodiazepine withdrawal), endocrine disturbances (e.g., hyperthyroidism), life stressors, and, once again, genetic/epigenetic interactions. The epigenetic disturbances underlying anxiety (and depression) appear to be rooted, in many cases, to emotional trauma.[3-5] These disturbances can result from traumas experienced during adulthood, childhood, *in utero* (in the womb), and may even be the result of ancestral traumas, as discussed in Chapter 20.[6]

Psychedelic medicines, like MDMA and psilocybin, have shown great promise in the treatment of anxiety disorders, including treatment-resistant PTSD and end-of-life anxiety in terminal cancer patients.[7-11] Current animal and human research indicates that ayahuasca, and its component alkaloids, can similarly be helpful in the treatment of anxiety disorders.[9,11] That has certainly been our experience at the center.

For nearly thirty years, Adam had been on one treatment or another for his anxiety disorder. Over email, we discussed his medical treatment. In preparation for his visit to Nihue Rao, he was planning to wean off of his anxiety medication Xanax (alprazolam: once more, a benzodiazepine in the same family as Valium). He had planned to be off of this medication for a full three weeks before coming to the center. One must wean off of benzodiazepines carefully. Stopping them too rapidly can lead to dangerous withdrawal symptoms, including seizures. I advised him to discuss this plan with his physician. Although this medication is not necessarily contraindicated with ayahuasca, we wanted him to be stable off of medication for the sake of his plant diet, and to prevent any possible interactions with any other plants involved. After a few email exchanges, Adam scheduled his visit to Nihue Rao, preparing himself accordingly. He brought his medication in case of emergency, but was committed to working through his symptoms without it.

Concerning his psychiatric history, Adam told me, "I've had anxiety since I was about twenty-six. I mean, we're talking almost thirty years that I've had anxiety, and depression related to anxiety. I tried a lot of stuff over the course of those years. Everything from cognitive therapy to medications. I have tried every antidepressant that there was. I'm just not a big pharmaceutical guy, but I tried a bunch of stuff . . . never worked. The only thing that ever really worked for me, and it was only partially, was Xanax, as needed.

"I was on a pretty low dose and it was as needed, so I didn't take it four times a day. I probably did take it five days of the week, though. It was kind of like a crutch. I'd have it with me in the car or a tablet in my pocket just in case I ever needed it. I never really thought that I was hooked on that [stuff] (Xanax is known to be addictive), but I do definitely think I had some withdrawal symptoms when I was down in Peru. I know it's a really hard one to kick. Yeah, I was on that medicine for more than twenty years.

Going to Peru was "kind of like my last straw. I felt like I was sick. A guy just going through life on the sidelines. I wanted to experience life again. Anxiety has been holding me back. I've got a lot of fear. I want to work through all that stuff. I was in a place in my life I've never been before. I was so willing . . . because I'd tried so many different things."

In addition to therapy and medications, Adam had also tried acupuncture. When he was younger, he had practiced yoga and meditation regularly, but now was no longer motivated to keep these practices going. As he told me, "I got to a point in my life where I just felt sick, and I wasn't doing anything. That's why I needed something drastic. That's why I chose ayahuasca, let's go down there and shake it up."

At the time, Adam was living alone in the Southern United States with his dog. He had been divorced for several years. His ex-wife lives in Germany, her native country, with their daughter. Concerning his career, Adam was in a transition, having previously worked as a filmmaker and professor.

I missed Adam's visit to the center, but we stayed in touch, and I interviewed him after he got home, about three weeks after his ten-day stay.

"My intentions were basically, on the sensible level, to get rid of the anxiety, get rid of the fear, depression in my life, and then, secondarily, figure out what I want to do with my life. Get some direction. Looking for a do over, basically. That's how I approached it, that's how I went into it."

He arrived at Nihue Rao in the usual way. He was happy to meet a group of interesting and friendly people there, *pasajeros* and staff. He went over his intentions with Ricardo and the team, and was prescribed a *vegetalista* diet with piñon blanco (the scientific doctor and bringer of light).

In our phone interview, I asked Adam about his ceremonies. He reviewed his journal notes as we discussed his experience.

"I read a few books on the topic, but nobody can prepare you for it. Every ceremony except the last one was just really [butt]-kicking. They were brutal. The first two ceremonies were so cathartic. Like I said, nothing could've prepared me.

"These are my notes from the first ceremony: Lots of purging, many visions, saw some animated cartoon characters come into the light. My mouth and throat transformed into the mouth of an anaconda and I exhaled my fears and pain. Snakes went in my nose and down my throat and cleaned out my entire body. I saw my fears and worked on healing relationships with my ex-wife and all of my old girlfriends. I gained a lot of clarity. I had a bad relationship with my ex-wife for all those years, and the medicine told me that my ex-wife had a miscarriage, and it broke her, and that's why she became bitter and hard towards me. I [could then feel] love and compassion for her.

"I had blocked that. I remembered now that she had a miscarriage before my daughter was born, but I had totally blocked that out. The thing was, that ceremony, I went through so much stuff that I had blocked, you know? It really was an autobiographical experience.

"The first night was taking me through everything. I would be so tired, I'd be on my mat, rocking back and forth. I would work and then I'd lie down and then mama [ayahuasca] would say, 'All right you got to get up again. We've got to go work some more' and I'm like, 'Ah, man, I just want to rest.' I just kept working through it, working through it. After the end of the first ceremony, I felt better, but fractured. I was between my old sick self and my new healed self. It was really working deep and it was a little scary.

"My second ceremony, same thing, just more cleansing, going deeper and deeper, again, I was seeing visions and we were working on my fear. Rolando [who had come to work at Nihue Rao] was singing and I was listening to him and to the shaman on his left."

At some point in the night, Adam was brought up to receive his personal healing song from Rolando. The helper reminded Rolando of Adam's goals, that he wanted to work on his fears.

Adam recalled the experience: "Rolando's icaro was very powerful, like an exorcism. I saw a vision of an older warrior chief that was exorcising the fear out of me. His voice rising higher and higher in intensity. I saw red flames in front of me, like a bellows blowing a furnace. With every verse of his icaro, the intensity rose. The fire grew stronger and brighter, and the color changed from red to orange and then to gold. I grew stronger and stronger in size. The icaro was transforming me from a fearful little man into a brave warrior leader. My entire body was shaking violently. [After the song] Rolando reached out and put his fingers on my head and blew mapacho smoke over me.

"I went from fearful to fearless. I saw myself as a young, fit warrior. I sat tall on my horse and became the leader in a ceremony of my people. It just felt so right to surrender to the medicine. It was just super, super intense.

"After the ceremony, I asked the guy sitting next to me, 'Who was the old guy that was singing next to Rolando, on his left?'

"He said, 'There was nobody to his left.' It was a fricking vision . . . crazy. That was the second ceremony."

Between the second and third ceremonies, Adam developed tremors. He explained, "My head would involuntarily shake from time to time. I thought the ayahuasca had unlocked some hidden disease, like

Parkinson's. My grandmother had that. My head would just uncontrollably shake. I was terrified and regretful about having gone to Peru. The shaman said it was normal, not to worry."

Adam was too far out from his medications to be in withdrawals; he was experiencing some kind of mystical energetic release. Traditionally, this kind of release is considered normal within the context of a master plant diet. Beyond the ceremonies, the piñon blanco and the ayahuasca were, as we say, still working on him. This shaking was releasing energy from his emotional body. The master plants direct traditional Shipibo healing, continuing the work in the day and off nights, helping peel back layer after layer, in preparation for ceremony.

Adam's third ceremony was heavy and overwhelming. His notes read, "All I saw was darkness, a sense of dread, heavy burden, body was shaking uncontrollably to the icaros. First I was sweating buckets, then I was freezing cold. Curled up in a fetal position and praying for the shaking and terror to go away. I couldn't see any visions or light. Everything was just dark and heavy.

"After the ceremony, my senses were hyper acute. I was very unstable and needed help going back to my tambo. That lasted into the next day. I could hear a pin drop. If anybody spoke, it was like nails on a chalkboard. I was just very on edge the whole time.

"In fact, I was so freaked out that I talked with Emilie and told her I didn't want to drink anymore [ayahuasca]." Emilie reassured Adam and reminded him that he was under no obligation to drink ayahuasca. The treatment team simply requested that Adam come to ceremony to receive his icaros.

Adam continued his diet and sat through his fourth ceremony without drinking. This is quite common in traditional Shipibo healing. Once someone is connected to the process, even without drinking ayahuasca, they often still have a mystical experience in ceremony. Although he did not drink, Adam felt shaky throughout the night. He was eventually called up for his song with Pedro, a visiting Shipibo shaman. Adam was so unsteady on his feet that he needed assistance to walk over to where Pedro was sitting.

Adam's Anxiety and the Calming Power of Compassion    229

"I didn't drink but I still had visions and felt the effects. I was moving to the music. My body was like a string puppet being moved back and forth and side to side. Pedro's icaro was very strong," he recalled. Pedro was singing in Shipibo, but Adam seemed to understand the words and the message, which penetrated into his body and soul. Through the icaro, Adam understood that although progress had been made, there was still more fear to clean.

"In the middle of the song, I reached up to my head and pulled off my false self, [revealing] a light being radiating love and life. A smile came to my face which spread from ear-to-ear. I felt so completely relaxed and also so very tired. My body was light as air. After my icaro, I went back to my mat and fell into a deep, deep sleep. After the ceremony finished, I went back to my tambo and again fell into a deep sleep, like I haven't slept in years. That was amazing and that was without drinking."

Adam then rested through the weekend, continuing his diet and his healing process with piñon blanco. On Monday, he entered his fifth ceremony. He decided to once again drink ayahuasca, reducing his dose. It turned out to be another night of intense cleaning, cleansing energies from his own life and from beyond.

"All night, cleaning and purging. First I purged my fearful cells, then I cleaned my insides completely. After this life was clean, I cleaned my past lives and purged out all the darkness I could find. My cleaning was very physical and I purged violently. When my past lives were clean, I continued to purge for the people who were not able to purge.

"I would talk to the ayahuasca, 'Why?' I'm clean and yet I'm still purging and she's like, 'You have to purge for those people that can't purge,' and I said, 'Okay.' I experienced their fears and trauma and purged it all. I felt such compassion for them, for people who could not purge because they were too old or infirm to do so. The icaros really moved me, and again my body rocked and shook to their vibration. I surrendered completely but was so exhausted by the end of it. I also connected briefly with my master plant piñon blanco. It was hard to keep focus for more than a few fleeting moments."

On the next night, his sixth and final ceremony, Adam cut his dose back further. After so much intensity, he longed for a milder experience.

"For the sixth ceremony, my intention was just really about my future. You know, they tell you not to expect anything. I learned that ayahuasca gives you what you need, not necessarily what you want. I was hoping to get some vision of me in my future career or relationship or something. It didn't really work that way. It was the least demanding ceremony. I was high, but I wasn't as high. I focused on the icaros, moved my head to the music. The experience was much less intense. When I asked what my future would be, I saw a picture of a blank whiteboard, you know, what you write on with magic markers.

"What came was me in front of this whiteboard, and the message was blank slate, clean slate, which meant, I write my own future both in love and career. My body was pure white-light energy. I'm not carrying any baggage with me into the future. The answer was, your future is what you make it. You don't have any baggage. You're clean, but, you know, I'm not telling you what your future is. You make it yourself."

Many *pasajeros* come to ceremony hoping to glimpse their mysterious future, their future love life and/or career. For the Shipibos, though, clearing up your past and present is much more valuable. By clearing up your mind, emotions, and body, you can more clearly sense your heart's desire. Once unblocked and healthy, once maladaptive programs are addressed, a more practical internal guidance is revealed. A healthy emotional body can help us to sense that which is beyond our mind's understanding. We learn to sense what drives us presently and why. Over time, this sense guides us to what we are called to do.

To some degree, Adam experienced this kind of clearing. As he told me, "Ayahuasca didn't give me what I wanted, it gave me what I needed. It cleaned out all of those blockages. Here we are now. I left there on the tenth of February, so it's been three weeks or so since I left. I'm a guy that had anxiety every day, whether I took medicine or not. I'm not taking any medicine now since I left. I'm still not taking it. I don't even take an aspirin now."

"I sleep really well now. I was sick for about a week when I came back. I still don't know whether I had malaria or not, but I was so weak for about a week, and I had a really bad hacking cough for about ten days [and now all of that is better]. It's definitely getting better now. [This treatment] saved my life, because it just really rebooted me. I guess that's how I can put it."

I asked him if he felt like he got what he was looking for. He replied, "100 percent Yes."

As the days went on, though, he noticed that the afterglow began to fade. As with Mike, who came back feeling healed, there was still more work to do. As Ricardo would say, this was Adam's first process.

"The day I left, I was sort of [in a state] of hyperrealism, you know, where everything was kind of acute. I felt like I was walking on air. My body had no weight to it. I was just really joyful. I was somewhere between worlds. I wasn't in the physical world and I wasn't completely in the spirit world. It was a bit unsettling and it was kind of cool.

"I'll also be honest with you, though. Now I've been back for, you know, several weeks, and the experience changes," he added. Things became challenging again; once he returned to our "messed up world," as he put it, his fears began to return.

"Now I'm back, I'm fully entrenched, but the anxiety is not the same. I start to focus too much about stuff, what am I going to do to make money, this and that. I can start to feel anxious again, but it's not the same," he said.

He still had anxious tendencies and would still get triggered, but not like before. Maladaptive programming had been altered, but Adam was still vulnerable.

Adam was struggling to integrate his Amazonian experiences with his American life. Alone, this was more difficult. "I went by myself, but obviously everybody there is connected because they've got a similar goal, they have a similar thought process, they're open to the medicine. Spiritually you're on the same path. Then coming back, you know, I come back to living by myself again, with my dog, kind of isolated. I have friends, but not everybody is open to the experience. It would be nice to have a local community that you can share that with, you know? We started a Facebook group and people have shared a little bit, but mostly just pictures. I've been in touch with a couple of people and we check in with each other."

As shamanic healer Malidoma Somé says, human beings need connection: connection to community, to nature, and to spirit. Adam had been through a significant cleanse, but once again he was alone and unsure about what to do with himself. Things were slipping.

He returned to his meditation practice and hoped to connect to a like-minded spiritual community. As Ricardo often says, Adam would need to "take good care of his medicine," meaning the medicinal energies he gained from the plants.

I checked in with him once more in July of 2016. His anxiety was back. He was managing his symptoms without medication which, after twenty years, was a significant improvement, but he was not healed. Fortunately, he had not lost all hope, but he needed more help. We spoke for a while and I learned that he had not followed up on his ayahuasca homework. He had not talked with his ex-wife about the miscarriage he saw in the visions. I encouraged him to reach out to her. I felt he needed to work on becoming more compassionate. Often, spiritual healing happens in stages.

As he considered his next moves, I put him in touch with someone who could help him integrate his experiences, someone who understands plant medicine and could offer him ongoing support and guidance. Adam continues to meditate and is now scheduling his next visit to Nihue Rao, for more cleansing and clearing. Hopefully he can plug into a supportive community soon, one that can help him find his way toward wellness.

Although the ayahuasca did not show Adam his future, she did give him a few ideas about what to work on. In the mystery of life, there are stepping stones. Once you step to the next stone, a new set of possibilities is revealed. This is how we progress down the spiritual path. Entering medical school, for example, I never imagined that I would one day study Shipibo shamanism in Peru. But stone by stone, I made my way down the Fellowship of the River, and just like Adam, my journey continues.

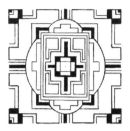

# CHAPTER 24

# The Role of Spiritual Healing in Modern Healthcare

I had sent him (an unnamed friend) my small book (*Future of Illusion*) that treats religion as an illusion, and he answered that he entirely agreed with my judgment upon religion, but that he was sorry I had not properly appreciated the true source of religious sentiments. This, he says, consists in a peculiar feeling, which he himself is never without, which he finds confirmed by many others, and which he may suppose is present in millions of people. It is a feeling which he would like to call a sensation of "eternity," a feeling of something limitless, unbounded—as it were, "oceanic." This feeling, he adds, is a purely subjective fact, not an article of faith.

—Sigmund Freud, *Civilization and Its Discontents*

And the path beyond the ordinary mind, all the great wisdom traditions have told to us, is through the heart.

—Sogyal Rinpoche, *The Tibetan Book of Living and Dying*

As I am finishing this book, I am heading down to South America once again, visiting family in Colombia on my way to Nihue Rao Centro Espiritual. This next two-month stint will mark the end of the Fellowship of the River. At the end of this year in 2016, I will step down as a business partner at Nihue Rao. As I plan to spend less time at the center, I cannot continue to manage things there. You can't really fly two kites, as they say. Perhaps I can continue to help as a consultant, but the time has come for me to find new ways to put my training into practice. For now, most importantly, I want to share some of what I have learned.

The Fellowship of the River has been an amazing adventure and a powerful medical education, one that has taught me a great deal about the value of spiritual healing. It is clear to me now, through working with hundreds of *pasajeros*, that in order to be healthy, humans need to be connected *to* and at peace *with* their environments, their communities, themselves, and the feeling in their hearts. It is through the heart that we come to know the subjective fact of oceanic boundlessness. Through the heart, we come to know spirit. We feel it, even if our minds cannot grasp it. Spirit is memories and spirit is possibilities. Spirit touches the flesh and is as real as heartache and joy. Spiritual dis-ease makes us sick, and spiritual healing helps us to become well.

I respect modern science and those who hold to its teachings as if it were their religion. I simply ask for that same respect, for my beliefs, and my interpretation of the current evidence. The Fellowship of the River has brought me to a new medical philosophy. Unlike the one I was exposed to in my allopathic training, this new philosophy does not ask me to deny my heart or soul; on the contrary, it demands that I acknowledge the emotional and spiritual dimensions of human health. In these times, we are dealing with an epidemic of soul sickness, i.e., spiritual illness. In order to adequately address this flood of spiritual maladies, we must expand our medical and cultural paradigms. At the very least, we must expand our capacity to identify and treat emotional illness.

As many medical and spiritual traditions have indicated, mind and body are paired. The emotional body (the PNEI network) helps to bridge mind and body. This emotional body has its own pair, the energy body, that which connects to spirit. The emotional body is a portal to energetic realms, connecting mind-body to spirit. This portal works both ways. We can approach the emotional body from the spiritual realms, healing the body through mystical techniques. In the other direction, the emotional body helps us to access the spiritual, and a healthier emotional body allows for greater access to mystical awareness.

When we neglect the emotional body, we compromise our access to the larger mystery. Such neglect, at an institutional level, breeds a society with limited access to personally meaningful and spiritually significant experiences. Cut off from inspiration, we are left to find emotional stimulation through material pursuits. This materialism often leaves us feeling disappointed. In this disappointment, we encourage one another to ignore how we feel about things, our relationships, our jobs, our culture, and our environment. At a personal level, neglect of the emotional body promotes disease like Russ's PTSD, Maria's back pain, and Lisa's migraines. And when healthcare practitioners ignore the underlying causes of this disease, emotional trauma (childhood trauma, war trauma, etc.) and stressful living, healing is delayed. Along the way, in this ignorance, precious healthcare resources are drained ineffectively.

Spiritual plant medicines like ayahuasca, peyote, and the master plants, when used properly, can help us to make up some ground with these kinds of problems. These spiritual medicines can help to heal our emotional-energy bodies and subsequently our mind-bodies. As we've seen in the cases presented, these ancestral medicines can be particularly useful in treating disorders rooted in emotional and energetic dysfunction. Psychedelic medicines, when used properly, can also provide similar healing. Modern clinical research supports the promise of all of these medicines. In practice, spiritual plant medicines, like all forms of spiritual healing, are most beneficial when utilized within a larger context involving continued integration and support. This might mean continued follow-up with a professional therapist or, perhaps, continued spiritual practice within a supportive community.

Whether it is through spiritual plant medicines, psychedelic medicines, spiritual practice, or simply the practice of love, the role of spiritual healing in modern healthcare is to treat the emotional and spiritual (energetic) dimensions of disease. As Ricardo often says, if your illness is of an energetic nature, chemical and physical approaches like medications and surgery will not solve your problem. You're going to need a shaman, a spiritual healer.

Shamanic approaches interact with the energy body. In this way, shamanic approaches help to heal dysfunction in the emotional body. When approaching this kind of dysfunction, Western diagnostic techniques should be used to rule out identifiable causes of illness. If such analysis does not reveal any clear cause, but instead points to measurable dysfunction in multiple regions of the emotional body, one should consider a shamanic or other spiritual approach. Such approaches should be explored further in the treatment of problems like depression, PTSD, idiopathic chronic cough, psychosomatic pain, psoriasis and inflammatory skin conditions, addiction, migraine headaches, inflammatory bowel disease, and anxiety.

Spiritual well being is reflected in emotional health. This is where shamanism meets allopathic medicine. This is what I learned on the Fellowship of the River. In addition to introducing me to shamanic practice, the plants and the people of the Amazon rainforest taught me that:

1. In order to heal emotionally and spiritually, one must overcome rigid and narrow thinking, which likely involves DMN (Default Mode Network) dysfunction, and which closes our mind to our hearts. Although limited thinking patterns can function as protective mechanisms, in the long run, they end up blocking out unresolved past experiences and/or our present feelings, limiting our access to the emotional body. An unhealthy society can make matters worse by further reinforcing rigid and potentially harmful thinking. I was trapped in this kind of thinking while depressed in medical school. Out at the Peyote Church, the Spirit Walk reopened my mind to my heart and to the world around me.

2. Once we open our minds to our hearts, we regain access to our feelings and senses, and we become more aware of what needs to be healed in the emotional body (PNEI network), e.g., prior emotional traumas and unresolved emotional processes, etc. Russ, for example, was reminded to heal his familial relationships. Colleen was shown that she needed to love herself in ways that she had not learned as a child.

3. Unresolved stress and emotional trauma accumulate in the emotional body, and this manifests as allostatic load in the PNEI network. The energies and dynamic physiologic processes connected to unresolved stress and emotional trauma underlie what is traditionally described as spiritual illness. Unaddressed, these energies stay within us for decades, leading to physical illness, as we saw with Maria. In Karl's case, such energies led to a subconscious guilt that lingered within him for over seventy years. Through the spiritual processes of acceptance and forgiveness, these energies can be transformed.

4. Love is the acceptance of all things as they are without reservation.

5. These accumulated energies (akin to allostatic load) are reflected in epigenetic imprints in the PNEI network, which store memories of emotional trauma and stress. Just as this epigenetic software is influenced by stress and traumatic experiences, this software can also be influenced by mystical practices, like love, meditation, and, according to my hypothesis, shamanic icaros. We saw this with Sharon's response to meditation and plant shamanism, and with Lisa and Nathan's response to healing song. Spirit meets biochemistry at the epigenetic level. Incidentally, psychotherapy (which also works through an invisible emotional connection, i.e., limbic resonance) has also been shown to promote healing by inducing epigenetic changes.[1]

6. Spiritual healing, whether it involves shamanic plant medicine or other techniques, helps us to purge dysfunctional energies

(maladaptive programs) from our emotional body and guides us to transform them further through faculties of the soul (psyche): self-love, forgiveness, compassion, and gratitude. We saw this again and again, with Adam as he cleared fear and found compassion, and with Mike, who learned to reconcile his past and, for the first time, love himself.

7. In this process of emotional and spiritual healing, we gain further access to mystical experiences. Mystical experiences shape our sense of personal meaning and spiritual significance. They help us to open our minds further and connect to our hearts, allowing for further healing in the emotional body, inducing measurable improvements in the mind-body, i.e., the flesh.

The emotional body bridges the mind and body, and the heart is central to this whole apparatus—feeling, sensing, and interacting with mystical energies. Embodied consciousness exists within a larger mystery, beyond what our minds can understand. Paradoxically, access to this incomprehensible mystery is actually what allows us to make sense of things. Connection to the larger mystery gives us a sense of place and purpose in this life. This subjective connection to the boundless mystery, experienced through the emotional-energy body, is what we traditionally describe as faith.

I am not sure where my journey is headed next, but I have faith. Following my heart to the Amazon was the right move for me, and now my internal guidance is leading me elsewhere. I am very grateful for all of the time that I spent in the Amazon rainforest amidst all of its magic. I love the Amazon and I hope that we can protect this incredible resource and the powerful river that flows through it.

On this Earth, nature's magic is still alive. I am eternally grateful to my plant teachers, my shamanic teachers, to Cvita, and to everyone who has made this journey possible. And, although we don't always see eye-to-eye on everything, I am especially grateful to my friend and teacher Ricardo Amaringo. Thanks to him, I became a shaman. And I must, of course, send a special thank you to the ayahuasca, for all of the help.

As we once again make more space for the practice of spiritual plant medicine, we should remember to be both cautious and open-minded, like our ancestors. As ayahuasca and similar spiritual medicines find their place among the world's medical and spiritual healing traditions, we should not forget that, really, there is only one medicine, that which helps us to heal.


The End

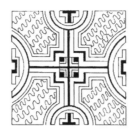

# Acknowledgments

This book would not have been possible without the support of my family: my mother and father, my brothers Mario and Camilo, my sisters-in-law Lilit and Martiza, my niece, and my nephews. I would like to thank them for all for their ever-present support. I would also like to express my gratitude to my grandparents, aunts, uncles, cousins, and all of my extended family and godchildren, including the illustrious Dirk Wiggins, whose crucial insight and support helped take this book to the next level. I would also like to offer heartfelt thanks to Dr. Hernando Garcia and his family.

I, of course, need to thank my shamanic family: Ricardo Amaringo, Cvita Mamic, Markus Drassl, and Martina Drassl, and all of the people who have dedicated themselves to helping people at Nihue Rao, with special thanks to Emilie Lescale and Philippe Favre. I must also thank my Arizona shamanic family: Anne Zapf, Matthew Kent, and their family. Thank you all for guiding me through the Fellowship of the River. I would have never made it without you. I would also like to extend a special thank-you to all of the long-term dieters at Nihue Rao; thank you for bringing the spirit to life.

I am eternally grateful to the Shipibo culture and all of the TAPM healers who guided my education, including: once more Ricardo

Amaringo, Rolando Tangoa Murayari, Miguel Muñoz, Julian Arevalo, Olivia Arevalo, Estela Pangoza, Wiler Noriega, Sulmira Vela, Celestina, Ronnie Vasquez, Marcelo Alvarez, Isabel Pinedo, Kestembetsa, Sonia Chuquimbalqui, Taita Juan Chindoy, Juan Flores, Percy Garcia, Maria Luisa, and all of the shamans I had the pleasure to work with at Nihue Rao, *Iraque*.

This work would not have been possible without the support of our Peruvian staff at Nihue Rao. Thank you for treating me like family. *Mil gracias,* thank you to each and every one of you from Llanchama, Iquitos, Pucallpa, and many other places.

I am also especially grateful to my plant teachers: ayahuasca, chacruna, coca, piñon blanco, bobinsana, ayahuma, ajo sacha, marosa, and peyote.

I would like to thank all of the visitors that I had a chance to meet and work with, whom we affectionately call the *pasajeros*, hailing from all over the world.

Of course, this project would not have been possible if it were not for the generosity and kindness of those special individuals who shared their healing stories for this book. Thank you for teaching me and inspiring me. God bless you.

Thank you to my official editor Caroline Pincus. I must admit that, once I read on her website that she had been described as "a shaman of words," I was pretty much sold, but then, once we spoke, I knew I had found a true ally for this project, so near and dear to my heart. Thank you for your brilliant insight and your kind friendship. When you weren't showing me how to improve my writing, you were pushing me to improve my writing. I could not have realized this project without you. Gracias. Thank you to Jeremy Narby for helping me find you.

I also need to thank all of my additional editors: my brother Mario, Michelle Chargois, and Ariel Whitworth, who helped me get this book off the ground, and to all of the people who helped guide this project further, including my brother Camilo, Maritza, Cvita, Martina, Markus, Dave S., my mom, Ian, and Kasi. Many blessings to all of you for your patience and consideration.

I would like to thank Dr. Gabor Maté for being a guiding example and an honest doctor, and for gracing this book with his thoughtful and precise foreword. I am very proud of this foreword, and I wish my father could see it, and I know he can, and I wish you and your family all of the best.

I would also like to thank Dr. Jeremy Narby and Dr. Alberto Villoldo for all of their inspiring work and for encouraging me to write this book. I must also thank pioneer and fellow ayahuasca researcher Dr. Dennis McKenna for his support.

Furthermore, I must give thanks to the faculty and staff of the following key educational institutions: the UCLA Department of Biology, the UCSD School of Medicine, St. Joseph's Hospital Family Medicine Residency, the UCLA Family Medicine Residency, the UCLA Center for East-West Medicine, the Pacific College of Oriental Medicine, the Scripps Center for Integrative Medicine, and the UCSD Department of Psychiatry. In particular, I would like to thank two key mentors, Dr. Sandra Daley and Dr. Paul Mills.

I would also like to thank several wonderful friends, colleagues, and loved ones for their special contributions to this adventure: Keyvan Hariri, Sabrina Sykes, Ken Kodama, R. Cahn, Rev. I. Trujillo, Dr. L. Miles, J. Felder, J. Brainin, K. Mohammadi, J. Dawley, D. Monaco, M. Casillas, Maria Yraceburu, M.A. Coveñas, the entire crew of Spaceship Earth (each and every one of you) with a special gracias to Bryon Hatcher, Russ Binicki, and Miguel Montiel, Dr. K. Eichelberger, Soi Bari, Flor, Sita, Chonon Yaca, Malidoma Somé, Mbali, Dr. S. Gomes, A. M. Coelho, Inti Munay, J. Rivera, Rosalia, J. Nuñez, C. Tanner, M. Watherston, S. Their, R. Feingold, U. Portocarerro, S.Vieira, Bia Labate, Charles Grob, Chris Kilham, Zoe Helene, Amber Lyon, T. Mathope, K. Hui, R. Bonakdar, Fred Kahn, A. Turner, C. Wells, James, E. Maupin, J. Harrison, R. P. Duncan, M. Muench, the Rev. John Robson, and many, many more.

Lastly, many thanks to all of the hardworking medical scientists and academic researchers out there; thank you for continuing to develop our knowledge base and for proving to me that biology, emotion, and spirituality belong in the same sentence.

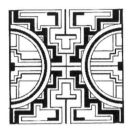

# Glossary

> . . . the scientist who charts the unexplored levels of organization to be found in nature, from the bizarre, paradoxical realms of quantum physics to the staggering vastness of the metagalaxy, has much in common with the shaman who journeys through the magical topography of the spirit-world.
>
> —Dennis McKenna and Terence McKenna,
> *The Invisible Landscape*

**Abuta (*Cissampelos pariera*):** a woody rainforest vine referred to by some as the midwives' herb because of its longtime use in the treatment of all types of feminine ailments.

**Ajo sacha: (*Mansoa alliace*):** a rain-forest tropical shrub which smells of garlic. It is known for its spiritual and medicinal properties. Used traditionally in shamanic training and to treat physical aches and pains.

**Allostatic load:** stress-related wear and tear, measured through stress-induced physiologic changes.

**Ayahuasca (*Banisteriopsis caapi*):** a woody vine native to the Amazon basin, considered by many cultures to be sacred, usually ingested as a tea in combination with other native psychotropic plants.

**Ayahuasquero/a:** an individual dedicated to working with ayahuasca in shamanic ceremony.

**Ayahuma** (*Couroupita guianensis*): a tall, tropical tree which grows up to thirty- five meters high and is well-known for its large cannonball-like fruits as well as its large brightly colored flowers, blended with pink, red and purple; also utilized in shamanic training.

**Ayurveda:** traditional system of medicine with historical roots in the Indian subcontinent.

**Azucena** (*Liliam spp*): flowering rain-forest plant which grows from a bulb and is used in plant vomitive preparations.

**Beso de la novia** (*Psychotria poeppigiana*): a flowering plant of the Amazon, used in some medicinal and toxic preparations, a close cousin of the chacruna.

**Boa huasca** (*Monstera spp*): a reddish, woody vine known in the Shipibo tradition for its medicinal value in treating both male and female reproductive issues; also utilized in shamanic training.

**Bobinsana** (*Calliandra angustifolia*): a shrubby tree which produces beautiful, pink and reddish powderpuff-like flowers; also utilized in shamanic training. Outside of shamanism, bobinsana is used as an herbal medicine for a variety of ailments, including joint pain and rheumatism.

**Chacruna** (*Psychotria viridis*): a bush native to the Amazon basin, rich in dimethyltryptamine (DMT), the powerful hallucinogen responsible for inducing ayahuasca visions, considered a master (teacher) plant in Shipibo culture.

**Chiric sanango** (*Brunfelsia grandiflora*): a flowering shrub of the nightshade family with fragrant white and purple flowers. In the Shipibo tradition, the medicine of chiric sanango is believed to bring fortification to the joints and physical body (when dieted in traditional fashion); also utilized in shamanic training.

**Coca** (*Erythroxylum coca*): a highly regarded medicinal plant in traditional Andean culture, across Bolivia, Peru, Ecuador, and Colombia, and an extremely nutritious plant, rich in essential minerals and vitamins. The Inca (the advanced pre-Columbian civilization which had controlled much of Peru until the arrival of the Spanish conquistadors) considered coca to be the most sacred plant medicine.

**Curare:** a plant-based poison, a muscle paralyzer, made in a variety of forms by Amazonian tribes and used traditionally for hunting game.

**Default Mode Network (DMN):** Neural network in the brain, which is most active when a person is not focused on the outside world (most active when, for example, thinking about oneself, the past, or the future). Overactivity of certain regions of this network is correlated to decreased awareness of the outside world and the body (interoception/emotional awareness) and to narrow and repetitive thinking patterns. Such overactivity has also been correlated to certain mental health problems including depression, anxiety and addiction.

**Dimethyltryptamine (DMT):** powerful psychedelic compound of the tryptamine family.

**Emotional body:** the medium through which we experience emotion and feeling.

**Epigenetics:** the study of that which exists *upon* the genes. Epigenetics is the study of trait variations that result from external or environmental factors that switch genes on and off and affect how cells express genes. For example, epigenetics explores how external factors like diet and lifestyle can affect the expression of genes causing problems like diabetes, cancer, and Parkinson's disease. The study of the range of possible phenotypes from any give genotype.

**HPA axis:** hypothalamic pituitary adrenal axis, central element of the stress response system.

**Icaro:** traditional healing song of the *ayahuasquero/a* and a central component of the Shipibo ayahuasca ceremony. The plants teach the *ayahuasquero/a* his/her song.

**La dieta:** see Vegetalista.

**La selva:** Spanish, meaning "the jungle."

**Limbic regulation:** mood contagion or emotional contagion. Once resonating, our limbic systems influence and regulate one another. In long-term relationships, limbic regulation affects the development and stability of our personality and mood (as defined in *A General Theory of Love*, cited in Chapter 13).

**Limbic resonance:** the ability of two people to tune in to each other's internal world and share an emotional state. This happens by attuning emotionally to subconscious cues (through the eyes, face, tone of voice, etc.) that arise from the limbic system.

**Limbic revision:** the therapeutic alteration of personality through therapeutic limbic regulation.

**Limbic system:** the emotional processing center of the brain, comprised of several areas of the brain, including, for example, the amygdala, hypothalamus, and hippocampus.

**LSD:** lysergic acid diethylamide, currently being investigated as a psychedelic medicine.

**Maloka:** large roundhouse in the jungle, of traditional construction.

**Mapacho (*Nicotiana rustica*):** Amazonian black tobacco.

**Mareación:** Spanish, the experience of feeling dizzy or disoriented, used to describe the physical and psychological effects of the ayahuasca.

**MDMA:** 3,4-methylenedioxy-methamphetamine, currently under investigation as a psychedelic medicine.

**Neurogenic inflammation:** inflammation generated by the nervous system, in the absence of injury or infection. Often a sign of dysfunction in the PNEI network (emotional body), possibly due to unresolved emotional trauma.

**OCD:** Obsessive Compulsive Disorder, a mental-health problem in which obsessive thoughts lead to compulsive behaviors.

**Ojé (*Ficus insipida*):** tall, tropical tree native to Latin America that begins its growth as a climbing vine (also utilized in shamanic training). The latex of this tree is traditionally used for its anti-parasitic and purgative properties.

**Pasajero/a:** Spanish, meaning passenger. Term used by some shamans to refer to seekers travelling to Peru in order to experience TAPM.

**Peyote (*Lophophora williamsii*):** a small, spineless, slow-growing cactus native to Mexico and parts of the Southwestern United States that contains the psychedelic alkaloid mescaline. Without harming the plant, the top section of the cactus can be carefully harvested as what's called a "peyote button" for ceremonial use.

**Piñon blanco (*Jatropha curcas*):** a rain-forest shrub with large oily seeds. In the Shipibo tradition, the spirit of the master plant piñon blanco is believed to bring a very pure light to the heart and mind.

**Psychoneuroendocrine Immunologic Network (PNEI):** the complex network connecting the brain's psychology to the nervous system, endocrine system, and immune system; theorized to be the physical manifestation of the emotional body.

**Psychoneuroimmunology (PNI):** the study of the connection between human psychology, the nervous system, and the immune system.

**PTSD:** Post-Traumatic Stress Disorder, a chronic anxiety disorder, which develops after exposure to a traumatic event.

**Serotonin:** neurotransmitter that plays a significant role in mood, also known as 5-hydroxytryptamine (5-HT).

**Shipibo:** indigenous culture of the Peruvian Upper Amazon, originating from the Ucayali River Basin.

**Shitana:** Shipibo, meaning the dark energy of the plants.

**Soplar:** Spanish, meaning to blow.

**Soplos:** Spanish, meaning "blowings," used to describe shamanic exhalations believed to carry intentional energies.

**SSRI:** Selective Serotonin Reuptake Inhibitor, e.g., fluoxetine (Prozac).

**Stress-response system:** physiologic system within the body which reacts to short- and long-term stressors, responsible for the fight-or-flight response and responses to chronic stress (managed by the HPA axis).

**Susto:** Spanish, meaning a scare. *Susto* is a Latin-American concept in which a traumatic event causes such a fright that the soul, or part of the soul, is scared out of the body. This is more common in children who are particularly sensitive to such trauma.

**Tambo:** Peruvian Spanish, meaning jungle hut.

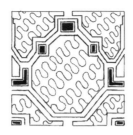

# References by Chapter

The indigenous shamans, who are known as taitas in Colombia, emphasize that yajé (ayahuasca) is not a "drug" but rather, a sacred plant which chastises (their own word) the drinker in order to bring about his reformation in every sense. In some cases, the harsh physical reactions to the brew do not result from a physical illness but point to a moral or emotional imbalance that expresses itself in bad conduct, negative thought, depression, and so forth.

—Jimmy Weiskopf, *Yajé (yagé): The New Purgatory,*
*Encounters with Ayahuasca*

## Chapter 1. The Fellowship of the River

1. Buhner S (2014). *Plant Intelligence and the Imaginal Realm*. Rochester, Vermont. Bear & Company.

## Chapter 3. The Wounded Healer

1. Puthran, et. al. Prevalence of depression amongst medical students: a meta-analysis. *Med Educ.* 2016 Apr;50(4):456-68.

2. Medscape, http://www.medscape.com/viewarticle/838437

# Chapter 4. Peyote Way

1. Halpern, JH. Hallucinogens and dissociative agents naturally growing in the United States. *Pharmacology & Therapeutics.* 2004;102:131-138.

2. El-Seedi, HR, et al. Prehistoric peyote use: Alkaloid analysis and radiocarbon dating of archaeological specimens of Lophophora from Texas. *Journal of Ethnopharmacology.* 2005 Apr;101:238-242.

3. Nichols, Dave E., Serotonin and the Past and Future of LSD. www.maps.org/news-letters/v23n1/v23n1_p20-23.pdf.

4. Vollenweider, FX, and M Kometer. The neurobiology of psychedelic drugs: implications for the treatment of mood disorders. *Nat Rev Neurosci.* 2010 Sep;11(9):642-51.

5. Amoroso, T. The Psychopharmacology of ±3,4 Methylenedioxymethamphetamine and Its Role in the Treatment of Post-Traumatic Stress Disorder. *J Psychoactive Drugs.* 2015 Nov-Dec;47(5):337-44.

6. Dos Santos, et al. Antidepressive, anxiolytic, and antiaddictive effects of ayahuasca, psilocybin, and lysergic acid diethylamide (LSD): a systematic review of clinical trials published in the last 25 years: Antidepressive effects of ayahuasca, psilocybin, and LSD. *Ther Adv Psychopharmacol.* 2016 Jun;6(3):193-213.

7. Rucker, JJ, et al. Psychedelics in the treatment of unipolar mood disorders: a systematic review. *J Psychopharmacol.* 2016 Dec;30(12):1220-1229.

8. McKenna, DJ. Clinical investigations of the therapeutic potential of ayahuasca: rationale and regulatory challenges. *Pharmacol Ther.* 2004 May;102(2):111-29. Review.

9. Halpern, JH, et al. Psychological and cognitive effects of long-term peyote use among Native Americans. *Biol Psychiatry.* 2005 Oct 15;58(8):624-31.

10. Bouso, JC, et al. Personality, psychopathology, life attitudes, and neuropsychological performance among ritual users of Ayahuasca: a longitudinal study. *PLoS One.* 2012;7(8):e4241.

11. Johansen, P and TS Krebs. Psychedelics not linked to mental health problems or suicidal behavior: a population study. *J Psychopharmacol.* 2015 Mar;29(3):270-9.

12. Strassman, RJ, et al. Dose-response study of N,N-dimethyltryptamine in humans. II. Subjective effects and preliminary results of a new rating scale. *Arch Gen Psychiatry.* 1994 Feb;51(2):98-108.

13. Ross, S, et .al. Rapid and sustained symptom reduction following psilocybin treatment for anxiety and depression in patients with life-threatening cancer: a randomized controlled trial. *J Psychopharmacol.* 2016 Dec;30(12):1165-1180.

14. Griffith, Roland R, et al. Psilocybin produces substantial and sustained decreases in depression and anxiety in patients with life-threatening cancer: A randomized double-blind trial. *J Psychopharmacol.* 2016;30(12);1181–1197.

15. Johnson, MW, et al. Pilot study of the 5-HT2AR agonist psilocybin in the treatment of tobacco addiction. *J Psychopharmacol.* 2014 Nov;28(11):983-92.

# Chapter 5. Mind, Feeling, and Faith

1. Spreng, RN, et al. The common neural basis of autobiographical memory, prospection, navigation, theory of mind, and the default mode: a quantitative meta-analysis. *J Cogn Neurosci.* 2009 Mar;21(3):489-510.

2. Van Wingen, GA, et al. Short-term antidepressant administration reduces default mode and task-positive network connectivity in healthy individuals during rest. *Neuroimage.* 2014 Mar;88:47-53.

3. Posner, J, et al. Antidepressants normalize the default mode network in patients with dysthymia. *JAMA Psychiatry.* 2013 Apr;70(4):373-82.

4. Hahn, A, et al. Differential modulation of the default mode network via serotonin-1A receptors. *Proc Natl Acad Sci U S A.* 2012 Feb 14;109(7):2619-24.

5. Carhart-Harris, RL, et al. The entropic brain: a theory of conscious states informed by neuroimaging research with psychedelic drugs. *Front Hum Neurosci.* 2014 Feb 3;8:20.

6. Bouso, JC, et al. Long-term use of psychedelic drugs is associated with differences in brain structure and personality in humans. *Eur Neuropsychopharmacol.* 2015 Apr;25(4):483-92.

7. Palhano-Fontes, F, et al. The psychedelic state induced by ayahuasca modulates the activity and connectivity of the default mode network. *PLoS One.* 2015 Feb 18;10(2).

8. Dos Santos, et al. Antidepressive, anxiolytic, and antiaddictive effects of ayahuasca, psilocybin, and lysergic acid diethylamide (LSD): a systematic review of clinical trials published in the last 25 years: Antidepressive effects of ayahuasca, psilocybin, and LSD. *Ther Adv Psychopharmacol.* 2016 Jun;6(3):193-213.

9. Sanches, RF, et al. Antidepressant Effects of a Single Dose of Ayahuasca in Patients with Recurrent Depression: A SPECT Study. *J Clin Psychopharmacol.* 2016 Feb;36(1):77-81.

10. Moreno, F, et al. Safety, tolerability, and efficacy of psilocybin in 9 patients with obsessive-compulsive disorder. *J Clin Psychiatry.* 2006 Nov;67(11):1735-40.

11. Domínguez-Clavé, E,et al. Ayahuasca: Pharmacology, neuroscience, and therapeutic potential. *Brain Res Bull.* 2016 Sep;126(Pt 1):89-101.

12. Soler, J, et al. Exploring the therapeutic potential of Ayahuasca: acute intake increases mindfulness-related capacities. *Psychopharmacology* (Berl). 2016 Mar;233(5):823-9.

13. Taylor, VA, et al. Impact of meditation training on the default mode network during a restful state. *Soc Cogn Affect Neurosci.* 2013 Jan;8(1):4-14.

14. Garrison, KA, et al. Meditation leads to reduced default mode network activity beyond an active task. *Cogn Affect Behav Neurosci.* 2015 Sep;15(3):712-20.

15. Griffiths, R, et al. Mystical-type experiences occasioned by psilocybin mediate the attribution of personal meaning and spiritual significance 14 months later. *J Psychopharmacol.* 2008 Aug;22(6):621-32.

16. Griffiths, RR, et al. Psilocybin occasioned mystical-type experiences: immediate and persisting dose-related effects. *Psychopharmacology.* 2011 Dec;218(4):649-65.

# Chapter 6. Tukuymanta

1. Davis, Wade (2010). *One River: Explorations and Discoveries in the Amazon Rainforest,* New York. Simon & Schuster.

2. Beyer, Stephan (2009) *Singing to the Plants: A Guide to Mestizo Shamanism in the Upper Amazon,* Albuquerque, New Mexico. University of New Mexico Press.

# Chapter 7. Responsible Practice

1. Carhart-Harris, RL, et al. The entropic brain: a theory of conscious states informed by neuroimaging research with psychedelic drugs. *Front Hum Neurosci.* 2014 Feb 3;8:20.

2. Szmulewicz, AG, et al. Switch to mania after ayahuasca consumption in a man with bipolar disorder: a case report. *Int J Bipolar Disord.* 2015 Feb 24;3:4.

# Chapter 8. Treating PTSD aboard Spaceship Earth

1. American Psychiatric Association (2013). *Diagnostic and Statistical Manual of Mental Disorders* (5th ed.). Arlington, VA: American Psychiatric Publishing. pp. 271–280.

2. Rauch, SA, et al. Prolonged exposure for PTSD in a Veterans Health Administration PTSD clinic. *J Trauma Stress.* 2009 Feb;22(1):60-4.

3. Chard, KM, et al. A comparison of OEF and OIF veterans and Vietnam veterans receiving cognitive processing therapy. *J Trauma Stress.* 2010 Feb;23(1):25-32.

4. Lancaster, CL, et al. Post-Traumatic Stress Disorder: Overview of Evidence-Based Assessment and Treatment. *J Clin Med.* 2016 Nov 22;5(11).

5. Todd, E. The Value of Confession and Forgiveness According to Jung. *Journal of Religion and Health.* 1985 Spring 24(1):39-44.

6. Mausbach, BT, et al. A 5-year longitudinal study of the relationships between stress, coping, and immune cell beta(2)-adrenergic receptor sensitivity. *Psychiatry Res.* 2008 Sep 30;160(3):247-55.

7. Mausbach, BT, et al. Stress-related reduction in personal mastery is associated with reduced immune cell beta2-adrenergic receptor sensitivity. *Int Psychogeriatr.* 2007 Oct;19(5):935-46.

# Chapter 9. The Emotional Body

1. Palhano-Fontes, F, et al. The psychedelic state induced by ayahuasca modulates the activity and connectivity of the default mode network. *PLoS One.* 2015 Feb 18;10(2).

2. Renate, LEP, Reniersa, et al. Moral decision-making, ToM, empathy and the default mode network. *Biological Psychology.* Volume 90, Issue 3, July 2012, pp. 202–210.

3. Mausbach, BT, et al. The attenuating effect of personal mastery on the relations between stress and Alzheimer caregiver health: a five-year longitudinal analysis. *Aging Ment Health.* 2007 Nov;11(6):637-44.

4. Mausbach, BT, et al. The moderating effect of personal mastery and the relations between stress and Plasminogen Activator Inhibitor-1 (PAI-1) antigen. *Health Psychol.* 2008 Mar;27(2S):S172-9.

5. Roepke, SK, et al. Personal mastery is associated with reduced sympathetic arousal in stressed Alzheimer caregivers. *Am J Geriatr Psychiatry.* 2008 Apr;16(4):310-7.

6. Mausbach, BT, et al. A 5-year longitudinal study of the relationships between stress, coping, and immune cell beta(2)-adrenergic receptor sensitivity. *Psychiatry Res.* 2008 Sep 30;160(3):247-55.

7. Roepke, SK, et al. The moderating role of personal mastery on the relationship between caregiving status and multiple dimensions of fatigue. *Int J Geriatr Psychiatry.* 2009 Dec;24(12):1453-62.

8. Dennis, PA, et al. Examining the Crux of Autonomic Dysfunction in Posttraumatic Stress Disorder: Whether Chronic or Situational Distress Underlies Elevated Heart Rate and Attenuated Heart Rate Variability. *Psychosom Med.* 2016 Sep;78(7):805-9.

9. Daskalakis, NP, et al. Endocrine aspects of post-traumatic stress disorder and implications for diagnosis and treatment. *Endocrinol Metab Clin North Am.* 2013 Sep;42(3):503-13.

10. Lindqvist D, et al. Proinflammatory milieu in combat-related PTSD is independent of depression and early life stress. *Brain Behav Immun.* 2014 Nov;42:81-8.

11. Bouso, JC, et al. MDMA-assisted psychotherapy using low doses in a small sample of women with chronic posttraumatic stress disorder. *J Psychoactive Drugs.* 2008 Sep;40(3):225-36.

12. Mithoefer, MC, et al. The safety and efficacy of {+/-}3,4-methylenedioxymethamphetamine-assisted psychotherapy in subjects with chronic, treatment-resistant posttraumatic stress disorder: the first randomized controlled pilot study. *J Psychopharmacol.* 2011 Apr;25(4):439-52.

13. Mithoefer, MC, et al. Durability of improvement in post-traumatic stress disorder symptoms and absence of harmful effects or drug dependency after 3,4-methylenedioxymethamphetamine-assisted psychotherapy: a prospective long-term follow-up study. *J Psychopharmacol.* 2013 Jan;27(1):28-39.

14. Amoroso, T, and M Workman. Treating posttraumatic stress disorder with MDMA-assisted psychotherapy: A preliminary meta-analysis and comparison to prolonged exposure therapy. *J Psychopharmacol.* 2016 Jul;30(7):595-600.

15. Tamburini, I, et al. MDMA induces caspase-3 activation in the limbic system but not in striatum. *Ann N Y Acad Sci.* 2006 Aug;1074:377-81.

16. Giannaccini, G, et al. Short-term effects of 3,4-methylen-dioxy-metamphetamine (MDMA) on 5-HT(1A) receptors in the rat hippocampus. *Neurochem Int.* 2007 Dec;51(8):496-506.

17. Riba, J, et al. Increased frontal and paralimbic activation following ayahuasca, the pan-Amazonian inebriant. *Psychopharmacology (Berl).* 2006 May;186(1):93-8.

18. Domínguez-Clavé, E, et al. Ayahuasca: Pharmacology, neuroscience and therapeutic potential. *Brain Res Bull.* 2016 Sep;126(Pt 1):89-101.

# Chapter 11. The Placebo Effect and Unexplainable Chronic Cough

1. Brody, H (1999). The Doctor as Therapeutic Agent: A Placebo Effect Research Agenda. A. Harrington (ed.) *The Placebo Effect: An Interdisciplinary Exploration* (pp. 77-92). Cambridge, Massachusetts. Harvard University Press.

2. Faruqi, S, et al. On the definition of chronic cough and current treatment pathways: an international qualitative study. *Cough.* 2014 May 29;10:5.

3. Cornere, MM. Chronic cough: a respiratory viewpoint. *Curr Opin Otolaryngol Head Neck Surg.* 2013 Dec;21(6):530-4.

4. Ryan, NM, et al. Arnold's nerve cough reflex: evidence for chronic cough as a sensory vagal neuropathy. *J Thorac Dis.* 2014 Oct; 6(Suppl 7):S748-52.

5. Altman, KW, et al. Neurogenic cough. *Laryngoscope.* 2015 Jul;125(7):1675-81.

6. Black, PH. Stress and the inflammatory response: a review of neurogenic inflammation. *Brain Behav Immun.* 2002 Dec;16(6):622-53.

# Chapter 12. Healing Hidden Trauma

1. http://www.rain-tree.com/ubos.htm#.V2oldI5wQ6g.

2. http://www.raintree.com/abuta.htm#.V2oknY5wR0s.

3. Modell, A (2003). *Imagination and the Meaningful Brain.* Cambridge, Massachusetts. The MIT Press.

# Chapter 13. Ayahuasca, TAPM, and Limbic Healing

1. Lewis, T, F Amini, and R Lannon (2000). *A General Theory of Love.* New York. Vintage Books.

# Chapter 16. Treating Psoriasis Spiritually

1. Boehncke, WH, and MP Schön. Psoriasis. *Lancet.* 2015 Sep 5;386(9997):983-94.

2. Menter, A, et al. Guidelines of care for the management of psoriasis and psoriatic arthritis: Section 1. Overview of psoriasis and guidelines of care for the treatment of psoriasis with biologics. *J Am Acad Dermatol.* 2008 May;58(5):826-50.

3. Connor, CJ, et al. Exploring the Physiological Link between Psoriasis and Mood Disorders. *Dermatol Res Pract.* 2015.

4. Harvima, RJ, et al. Association of psychic stress with clinical severity and symptoms of psoriatic patients. *Acta Derm Venereol.* 1996 Nov;76(6):467-71.

5. Hunter, HJ, et al. Does psychosocial stress play a role in the exacerbation of psoriasis? *Br J Dermatol.* 2013 Nov;169(5):965-74.

6. Martín-Brufau, R, et al. Psoriasis lesions are associated with specific types of emotions. Emotional profile in psoriasis. *Eur J Dermatol.* 2015 Jul-Aug;25(4):329-34.

7. Leslie, KS, et al. Sulphur and skin: from Satan to Saddam! *J Cosmet Dermatol.* 2004 Apr;3(2):94-8.

8. Buske-Kirschbaum, A, et al. Blunted HPA axis responsiveness to stress in atopic patients is associated with the acuity and severeness of allergic inflammation. *Brain Behav Immun.* 2010 Nov;24(8):1347-53.

9. Liezmann, C, et al. Stress, atopy, and allergy: A re-evaluation from a psychoneuroimmunologic perspective. *Dermatoendocrinol.* 2011 Jan;3(1):37-40.

10. Cvitanović, H, and E Jancić. Influence of stressful life events on coping in psoriasis. *Coll Antropol.* 2014 Dec;38(4):1237-40.

11. McEwen, BS. Stress, adaptation, and disease. Allostasis and allostatic load. *Ann N Y Acad Sci.* 1998 May 1;840:33-44. Review. Overiew.

12. Juster, RP, et al. Allostatic load and comorbidities: A mitochondrial, epigenetic, and evolutionary perspective. *Dev Psychopathol.* 2016 Nov;28(4pt1):1117-1146. Overview.

13. Mauss, D, et al. The streamlined Allostatic Load Index: a replication of study results. *Stress.* 2016 Nov;19(6):553-558.

14. Verburg-van Kemenade, BM, et al. Neuroendocrine-immune interaction: Evolutionarily conserved mechanisms that maintain allostasis in an ever-changing environment. *Dev Comp Immunol.* 2017 Jan;66:2-23.

15. Maloney, EM, et al. Chronic fatigue syndrome and high allostatic load: results from a population-based case-control study in Georgia. *Psychosom Med.* 2009 Jun;71(5):549-56. CFS.

# Chapter 17. Healing the Hurt at the Center of Addiction

1. Thomas, G, et al. Ayahuasca-assisted therapy for addiction: results from a preliminary observational study in Canada. *Curr Drug Abuse Rev.* 2013 Mar;6(1):30-42.

2. Dos Santos, RG, et al. Antidepressive, anxiolytic, and antiaddictive effects of ayahuasca, psilocybin, and lysergic acid diethylamide (LSD): a systematic review of clinical trials published in the last 25 years. *Ther Adv Psychopharmacol.* 2016 Jun;6(3):193-213.

3. Labate, B, and C Cavnar, eds. (2013). *The Therapeutic Use of Ayahuasca.* Springer Science & Business Media.

4. Loizaga-Velder, A, and R Verres. Therapeutic effects of ritual ayahuasca use in the treatment of substance dependence—qualitative results. *J Psychoactive Drugs.* 2014 Jan-Mar;46(1):63-72.

5. Oliveira-Lima, AJ, et al. Effects of ayahuasca on the development of ethanol-induced behavioral sensitization and on a post-sensitization treatment in mice. *Physiol Behav.* 2015 Apr 1;142:28-36.

6. Nunes, AA, et al. Effects of Ayahuasca and Its Alkaloids on Drug Dependence: A Systematic Literature Review of Quantitative Studies in Animals and Humans. *J Psychoactive Drugs*. 2016 May 26:1-11.

7. Malenka, RC, EJ Nestler, and SE Hyman (2009). "Chapter 15: Reinforcement and Addictive Disorder." In Sydor, A, and RY Brown (2009). *Molecular Neuropharmacology: A Foundation for Clinical Neuroscience* (2nd ed.). New York. McGraw-Hill Medical. pp. 364–365, 375.

8. Murray, JE, et al. Basolateral and central amygdala differentially recruit and maintain dorsolateral striatum-dependent cocaine-seeking habits. *Nat Commun*. 2015 Dec 14;6:10088.

9. Ladrón de Guevara-Miranda, D, et al. Cocaine-conditioned place preference is predicted by previous anxiety-like behavior and is related to an increased number of neurons in the basolateral amygdala. *Behav Brain Res*. 2016 Feb 1;298(Pt B):35-43.

10. Rovaris, DL, et al. Corticosteroid receptor genes and childhood neglect influence susceptibility to crack/cocaine addiction and response to detoxification treatment. *J Psychiatr Res*. 2015 Sep; 68:83-90.

11. https://www.drugabuse.gov/publications/drugfacts/nationwide-trends.

12. Richards, WA (2002). Entheogens in the study of mystical and archetypal experiences. *Research in the Social Scientific Study of Religion*, 13: pp. 143-155.

13. Griffiths, RR, et al. Psilocybin can occasion mystical-type experiences having substantial and sustained personal meaning and spiritual significance. *Psychopharmacology (Berl)*. 2006 Aug;187(3):268-83; discussion 284-92.

14. Griffiths, RR, et al. Mystical-type experiences occasioned by psilocybin mediate the attribution of personal meaning and spiritual significance 14 months later. *J Psychopharmacol*. 2008 Aug;22(6):621-32.

15. Garcia-Romeu, A, et al. Psilocybin-occasioned mystical experiences in the treatment of tobacco addiction. *Curr Drug Abuse Rev*. 2014;7(3):157-64.

16. Hall, W, et al. The brain disease model of addiction: is it supported by the evidence and has it delivered on its promises? *Lancet Psychiatry*. 2015 Jan;2(1):105-10.

# Chapter 19. Lisa's Migraine Headaches and the Black Dragon

1. Smitherman, TA, et al. The prevalence, impact, and treatment of migraine and severe headaches in the United States: a review of statistics from national surveillance studies. *Headache*. 2013 Mar;53(3):427-36.

2. Schindler, EA, et al. Indoleamine Hallucinogens in Cluster Headache: Results of the Clusterbusters Medication Use Survey. *J Psychoactive Drugs*. 2015 Nov-Dec;47(5):372-81.

3. Borsook, D, et al. Understanding migraine through the lens of maladaptive stress responses: a model disease of allostatic load. *Neuron*. 2012 Jan 26;73(2):219-34.

4. Maleki, N, et al. Migraine: maladaptive brain responses to stress. *Headache.* 2012 Oct;52 Suppl 2:102-6.

5. Tietjen, GE, et al. Childhood Maltreatment in the Migraine Patient. *Curr Treat Options Neurol.* 2016 Jul;18(7):31.

6. Meggs, WJ. Neurogenic inflammation and sensitivity to environmental chemicals. *Environ Health Perspect.* 1993 Aug;101(3):234-8.

7. Roos-Araujo D, et al. Epigenetics and migraine: complex mitochondrial interactions contributing to disease susceptibility. *Gene.* 2014 Jun 10;543(1):1-7.

8. Malhotra, R. Understanding migraine: Potential role of neurogenic inflammation. *Ann Indian Acad Neurol.* 2016 Apr-Jun;19(2):175-82.

## Chapter 20. Epigenetics, Inheritable Stresses, and Release through Spiritual Healing

1. McGowan, PO. Epigenomic Mechanisms of Early Adversity and HPA Dysfunction: Considerations for PTSD Research. *Front Psychiatry.* 2013 Sep 26;4:110.

2. Kaminsky, Z, et.al. Epigenetic and genetic variation at SKA2 predict suicidal behavior and post-traumatic stress disorder. *Transl Psychiatry.* 2015 Aug 25; 5: e627.

3. McGowan, PO. Epigenetics in mood disorders. *Environ Health Prev Med.* 2008 Jan;13(1):16-24.

4. Sun, H, et al. Epigenetics of the depressed brain: role of histone acetylation and methylation. *Neuropsychopharmacology.* 2013 Jan;38(1):124-37.

5. Holloway, T, and J González-Maeso. Epigenetic mechanisms of Serotonin Signaling. *ACS Chem Neurosci.* 2015. Jul 15; 6(7): 1099–1109.

6. Smart, C, et al. Early life trauma, depression, and the glucocorticoid receptor gene—an epigenetic perspective. *Psychol Med.* 2015 Dec;45(16):3393-410.

7. Trowbridge, RM, and MR Pittelkow. Epigenetics in the pathogenesis and pathophysiology of psoriasis vulgaris. *J Drugs Dermatol.* 2014 Feb;13(2):111-8.

8. Deng, Y, et al. The Inflammatory Response in Psoriasis: A Comprehensive Review. *Clin Rev Allergy Immunol.* 2016 Mar 30.

9. Naomi A, et al. New Developments in Human Neurocognition: Clinical, Genetic, and Brain Imaging Correlates of Impulsivity and Compulsivity. *CNS Spectr.* 2014 Feb; 19(1): 69–89.

10. Eising, E, et al. Epigenetic mechanisms in migraine: a promising avenue? *BMC Med.* 2013; 11:26.

11. Weaver, IC. Epigenetic programming by maternal behavior and pharmacological intervention. Nature versus nurture: let's call the whole thing off. *Epigenetics.* 2007 Jan-Mar;2(1):22-8.

12. McCrory, E, et al. The Impact of Childhood Maltreatment: A Review of Neurobiological and Genetic Factors. *Front Psychiatry.* 2011; 2:48.

13. Suderman, M, et al. Conserved epigenetic sensitivity to early life experience in the rat and human hippocampus. *Proc Natl Acad Sci U S A.* 2012 Oct 16;109 Suppl 2:17266-72.

14. Provençal, N, et al. The signature of maternal rearing in the methylome in rhesus macaque prefrontal cortex and T cells. *J Neurosci.* 2012 Oct 31;32(44):15626-42.

15. Bellis, M, and A Zisk. The Biological Effects of Childhood Trauma. *Child Adolesc Psychiatr Clin N Am.* 2014 Apr;23(2):185–222.

16. Roos-Araujo, D, et al. Epigenetics and migraine; complex mitochondrial interactions contributing to disease susceptibility. *Gene.* 2014 Jun 10;543(1):1-7.

17. Tietjen, GE, et al. Childhood Maltreatment in the Migraine Patient. *Curr Treat Options Neurol.* 2016 Jul;18(7):31.

18. Bowers, ME, and R Yehuda. Intergenerational Transmission of Stress in Humans. *Neuropsychopharmacology.* 2016 Jan;41(1):232-44.

19. Klengel T. et.al. Models of Intergenerational and Transgenerational Transmission of Risk for Psychopathology in Mice. *Neuropsychopharmacology.* 2016 Jan;41(1):219-31.

20. Mathews, H, and L Witek Janusek. Epigenetics and Psychoneuroimmunology: Mechanisms and Models. *Brain Behav Immun.* 2011 Jan; 25(1):25–39.

21. Qi-Bing, X, et al. Design, synthesis, and biological evaluation of hybrids of β-carboline and salicylic acid as potential anticancer and apoptosis inducing agents. *Sci Rep.* 2016;6:36238.

22. Dusek, JA, et al. Genomic counter-stress changes induced by the relaxation response. *PLoS One.* 2008 Jul 2;3(7):e2576.

23. Black, DS, et al. Yogic meditation reverses NF-κB and IRF-related transcriptome dynamics in leukocytes of family dementia caregivers in a randomized controlled trial. *Psychoneuroendocrinology.* 2013 Mar;38(3):348-55.

24. Kaliman, P, et al. Rapid changes in histone deacetylases and inflammatory gene expression in expert meditators. *Psychoneuroendocrinology.* 2014 Feb;40:96-107.

25. Lee, H. Impact of Maternal Diet on the Epigenome during In Utero Life and the Developmental Programming of Diseases in Childhood and Adulthood. *Nutrients.* 2015 Nov;7(11):9492–9507.

26. St-Cyr, S, and PO McGowan. Programming of stress-related behavior and epigenetic neural gene regulation in mice offspring through maternal exposure to predator odor. *Front Behav Neurosci.* 2015 Jun 1;9:145.

27. Dias, BG, and KJ Ressler. Parental olfactory experience influences behavior and neural structure in subsequent generations. *Nat Neurosci.* 2014 Jan;17(1):89-96.

# Chapter 22. Nathan's Crohn's Disease: Mystical Reprogramming and the Healing of a Broken Heart

1. Stefanelli, T, et al. New Insights into Inflammatory Bowel Disease Pathophysiology: Paving the Way for Novel Therapeutic Targets. *Current Drug Targets*. 2008, 9(5): 413–8.

2. Goodhand, JR, et al. Mood disorders in inflammatory bowel disease: relation to diagnosis, disease activity, perceived stress, and other factors. *Inflamm Bowel Dis*. 2012 Dec;18(12):2301-9.

3. Walker, E, et al. The relationship of current psychiatric disorder to functional disability and distress in patients with inflammatory bowel disease. *Gen Hosp Psychiatry*. 1996 Jul;18(4):220-9.

4. Filipovic, BR, and BF Filipovic. Psychiatric comorbidity in the treatment of patients with inflammatory bowel disease. *World J Gastroenterol*. 2014 Apr 7;20(13):3552-63.

5. de Fontgalland, D, et al. The neurochemical changes in the innervation of human colonic mesenteric and submucosal blood vessels in ulcerative colitis and Crohn's disease. *Neurogastroenterol Motil*. 2014 May;26(5):731-44.

6. Münster, T, et al. Characterization of somatosensory profiles in patients with Crohn's disease. *Pain Pract*. 2015 Mar;15(3):265-71.

7. McDermott, E, et al. DNA Methylation Profiling in Inflammatory Bowel Disease Provides New Insights into Disease Pathogenesis. *J Crohns Colitis*. 2016 Jan;10(1):77-86.

8. Bai, AH, et al. Dysregulated Lysine Acetyltransferase 2B Promotes Inflammatory Bowel Disease Pathogenesis through Transcriptional Repression of Interleukin-10. *J Crohns Colitis*. 2016 Jun;10(6):726-34.

9. http://www.newstaco.com/2013/06/07/the-science-behind-susto.

# Chapter 23. Adam's Anxiety and the Calming Power of Compassion

1. http://www.mentalhealthamerica.net/conditions/anxiety-disorders.

2. Müller, MB, et al. Hypothalamic-pituitary-adrenocortical system and mood disorders: highlights from mutant mice. *Neuroendocrinology*. 2004 Jan;79(1):1-12.

3. Shimada-Sugimoto, M, et al. Genetics of anxiety disorders: Genetic epidemiological and molecular studies in humans. *Psychiatry Clin Neurosci*. 2015 Jul;69(7):388-401.

4. Tyrka, AR, et al. Methylation of the leukocyte glucocorticoid receptor gene promoter in adults: associations with early adversity and depressive, anxiety, and substance-use disorders. *Transl Psychiatry*. 2016 Jul 5;6(7): e848.

5. Nieto, SJ, et al. Don't worry; be informed about the epigenetics of anxiety. *Pharmacol Biochem Behav*. 2016 Jul-Aug;146-147:60-72.

6. Zheng, Y, et al. Gestational stress induces depressive-like and anxiety-like phenotypes through epigenetic regulation of BDNF expression in offspring hippocampus. *Epigenetics*. 2016 Feb;11(2):150-62.

7. Grob, CS, et al. Pilot study of psilocybin treatment for anxiety in patients with advanced-stage cancer. *Arch Gen Psychiatry*. 2011 Jan;68(1):71-8.

8. Mithoefer, MC, et al. Novel psychopharmacological therapies for psychiatric disorders: psilocybin and MDMA. *Lancet Psychiatry*. 2016 May;3(5):481-8.

9. Dos Santos, RG, et al. Antidepressive, anxiolytic, and antiaddictive effects of ayahuasca, psilocybin, and lysergic acid diethylamide (LSD): a systematic review of clinical trials published in the last 25 years. *Ther Adv Psychopharmacol*. 2016 Jun;6(3):193-213.

10. Ross, S, et al Rapid and sustained symptom reduction following psilocybin treatment for anxiety and depression in patients with life-threatening cancer: a randomized controlled trial. *J Psychopharmacol*. 2016 Dec;30(12):1165-1180.

11. Dos Santos, RG, et al. Antidepressive and anxiolytic effects of ayahuasca: a systematic literature review of animal and human studies. *Rev Bras Psiquiatr*. 2016 Mar;38(1):65-72.

# Chapter 24. The Role of Spiritual Healing in Modern Healthcare

1. Roberts, S, et al. HPA Axis related genes and response to psychological therapies: genetics and epigenetics. *Depress Anxiety*. 2015 Dec;32(12):861-70.

# Index

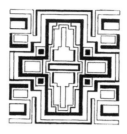

## F

family connections, 54–58
*Famished Road, The,* 1
faraway place, 39
fearful thoughts causing anxiety, 39
fibromyalgia, 104
*Ficus insipida,* 11
fight-or-flight response, 81–82
5-hydroxy*tryptamine* or 5-HT, 28
floral baths, 73–74
*Flora Medicinal de Colombia,* 46
Fluoxetine, 71
forgiveness, 76, 114, 131
Freud, Sigmund, 235

## G

Garcia, Darrio, 58
Garcia-Barrig, Hernando, 46–47, 56–58
gastrointestinal (GI) tract, 214
*General Theory of Love, The,* 117–118, 120–121
genetic factors for psoriasis, 147
Geriatrics Fellowship, 3
GI. *see* gastrointestinal (GI) tract
*Gods Must Be Crazy, The,* 36
Grand Rounds, 75–76
green energy, 181–182
Griffith, Dr. Roland, 172
*gringos,* 9
Gulf War, 70

## H

hallucinogenic drugs, 128–129
Harvard, 46, 57
headaches. *see* migraine headaches
healing spirit of nature, ayahuasca as, 8
Health Maintenance Organization (HMO), 44
Helene, Zoe, 106
herbal medicines, 45–46
hippies, 27–28
History Channel, 54
HMO. *see* Health Maintenance Organization (HMO)
Hoffman, Albert, 27, 55–56
Holocaust, 201
hopeless thoughts causing depression, 39
HPA. *see* hypothalamic-pituitary-adrenal (HPA) axis
human
    ayahuasca, senses to help with, 38–39
    basic necessities of, 21
    rights of, 36
hypersensitivity, 104
hypothalamic-pituitary-adrenal (HPA) axis, 82, 160, 215, 225
hypothalamus, 82

## I

IBD. *see* inflammatory bowel disease (IBD)
IBS. *see* irritable bowel syndrome (IBS)
ibuprofen, 184
icaro, 12–13, 15, 38, 48, 68, 73, 94, 141–143, 177, 179
identity, 119
Idiopathic Chronic Cough, 97
Imitre, 184
immune system, 81
Inca, 86
Indiana Jones, 10
infections, 146
inflammation. *see* neurogenic inflammation
inflammatory bowel disease (IBD), 213, 215
inherited epigenetics, 201
*Intelligence in Nature,* 195
*In the Realm of Hungry Ghosts: Close Encounters with Addiction,* 159–160
in utero trauma, 200
Iquitos, 9
Iraq, 79
irritable bowel syndrome (IBS), 213–214

## J

Japanese Zen meditation, 18
Johns Hopkins Medical School, 172–173
*Joy Luck Club, The,* 105
Jung, Carl, 76
*Jupiter Ascending,* 196

## K

Kalahari Desert, 37
Kamsá shamanism, 88
Kent, Rabbi Matthew, 30
Kilham, Chris, 106, 145
Kiowa natives, use of peyote, 55

## L

*la dieta,* 5
*la Madre* Ayahuasca, 7–8, 14, 61, 130
Lannon MD, Richard, 117
*la selva,* 13
Latin America, 58
Latino AIDS, 18
leaky gut syndrome, 147–148
learning diet, 85
Lewis MD, Thomas, 117
*libro,* 95
life-changing visions caused by ayahuasca, 8
*Liliam spp,* 11
limbic regulation, 120
limbic resonance, 120
limbic revision, 120–121
limbic system

Nihue Rao Centro Espiritual, 4, 9, 21
    ayahuasca, made in, 126–127
    development of, 90–92
*nihue rao* trees, 90–91
nonsteroidal anti-inflammatories (NSAIDs), 184
North American culture, 89
NSAIDs. *see* nonsteroidal anti-inflammatories
    (NSAIDs)

# O

Obsessive Compulsive Disorder (OCD)
    Default Mode Network, correlation with, 40
    psychedelic medicines for, 39–40
    repetitive thinking, symptom of, 39–40
OCD. *see* Obsessive Compulsive Disorder (OCD)
*ojé*, 11, 155, 205, 217
Okri, Ben, 1
*One River*, 54, 56–57
open-minded thinking, 39, 63
oppression, 36
optimism, 39
out-of-control inflammation caused by PTSD, 81
overactivity in Default Mode Network, 39–40

# P

Pacific College of Oriental Medicine (PCOM), 18
pain, psychosomatic, 118, 122
Palomares-Bernal, José "Pepe" M., 46, 56
paralysis, temporary, 53
Parkinson's disease, 188, 228–229
*pasajeros*, 10, 48–49, 59, 61, 90–91, 93–94, 99,
    107–108, 126, 129, 135
PCOM. *see* Pacific College of Oriental Medicine
    (PCOM)
Pegasus, 32
pena, 98–100
peripheral nervous system, 215
Personal Mastery Scale, 80–81
pessimism, 39
peyote, 2, 24, 237–238
    for depression, 26, 39
    Kiowa natives, use of, 55
    Native American Church, used by, 26
    Spirit Walk using, 25, 30–31, 34
    traditions using, 26
peyote button, 26
peyote cactus, 25–26, 37
*Peyote to LSD: The Psychedelic Odyssey*, 54
Peyote Way, 34, 37
Peyote Way Church of God, 25, 26, 29–30, 33, 36
phobias, 224
Phoenix Suns, 10, 15
physical body, 5
physiology, emotional, 81
piñon blanco *(Jatropha curcas)*, 126, 137–141, 155,
    205, 230
pituitary gland, 82

placebo effect, 94–102
*Placebo Effect, The*, 95
*Plants of the Gods, The*, 56
plaque psoriasis, 146
PNEI. *see* psychoneuro-endocrine-immunologic
    (PNEI) network
PNI. *see* psychoneuroimmunology (PNI)
poison, dart, 52–53
post-traumatic stress disorder (PTSD), 5
    abnormal adrenaline caused by, 81
    allostatic load associated with, 158
    anxiety, associated with, 81, 224–225
    cortisol levels during, 81
    defined, 70
    diagnosis of, 71
    emotional body, role in, 237
    emotional healing from, 81, 115
    emotional trauma, cause of, 81
    healing from, 80
    limbic system, control of, 118, 122
    out-of-control inflammation caused by, 81
    overreactive fight-or-flight response caused
        by, 81
    PNEI network, for healing of, 81
    psychedelic medicines for, 80, 82–83
    psychoactive medications for, 71
    shamanic plant medicine for, 63
    *vegetalista* diet for, 112–113
Prozac, 28, 71–72, 127
psilocybin, 27, 28, 40, 225
psoriasis, 146–156
    alternative medicine for, 147–148
    anxiety caused by, 155
    colonics for, 152
    defined, 146
    depression associated with, 146–147
    diagnosis of, 147
    emotional body and, 146–156
    emotional trauma related to, 148–150
    environmental factors triggering, 146–147
    genetic factors for, 147
    meditation for, 148
    neurogenic inflammation and, 104
    plaque, 146
    PNEI network for, 156
    types of, 146
psoriatic arthritis, 146
psychedelic medicine
    for addiction, 28, 29, 39–40
    for anxiety, 29, 39–40
    for depression, 29, 39–40
    Drug Enforcement Agency, classification of, 28
    history of, 27–29
    LSD as, 27–28
    for Obsessive Compulsive Disorder, 39–40
    for post-traumatic stress disorder, 29, 80,
        82–83
    for psychological trauma, 28
    religious use of, 29–34

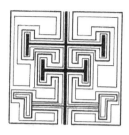

# About the Author

Dr. Joe Tafur is a Colombian-American family physician raised in Phoenix, Arizona. Throughout his medical career, he has been an integrative-medicine activist. As part of his exploration into holistic healthcare, he spent two years in academic research at the University of California, San Diego, department of psychiatry in a lab focused on mind-body medicine.

After his research fellowship, over a period of six years, he lived and worked in the Peruvian Amazon at the traditional healing center Nihue Rao Centro Espiritual. There he worked closely with master Shipibo shaman Ricardo Amaringo and trained in Traditional Amazonian Plant Medicine. At the center, Dr. Tafur completed traditional apprenticeship in ayahuasca shamanism. During those years at Nihue Rao, he assisted hundreds of individuals from all over the world as they went through traditional healing with Amazonian plant medicines and ayahuasca ceremony. He is both doctor and shaman.

Dr. Tafur is committed to healing work and to education. He is passionate about bridging the worlds of medical science and spiritual healing, and hopes to promote this work through lectures and educational programs. With his brother Mario and friends, he has founded the nonprofit organization Modern Spirit, which focuses on demonstrating the value of spiritual healing in modern healthcare through, among other avenues, educational programs for healthcare practitioners. If you are interested in supporting this work or having Dr. Tafur consult with your organization, please visit their website modernspirit.org. Dr. Tafur's independent work is further described at his personal website drjoetafur.com.

46811526R00178

Made in the USA
San Bernardino, CA
15 March 2017